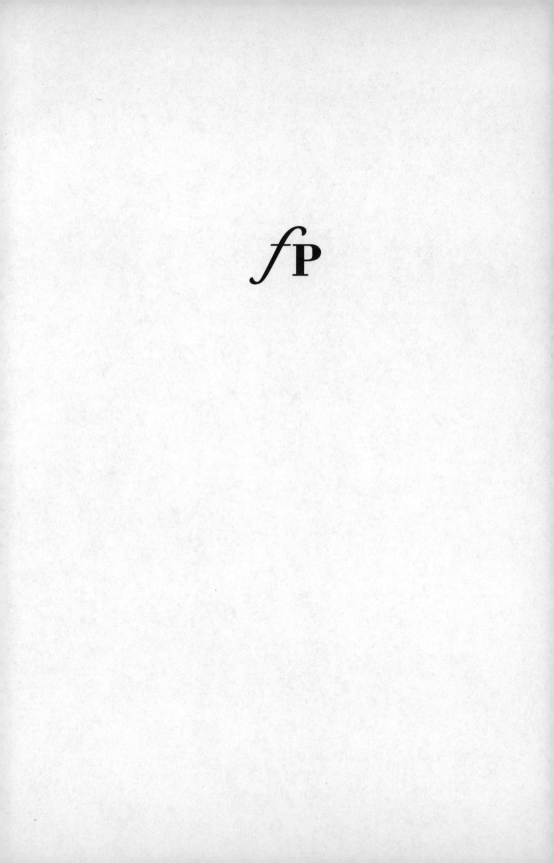

WHO THEY WERE

INSIDE THE WORLD TRADE CENTER DNA STORY:
THE UNPRECEDENTED EFFORT TO
IDENTIFY THE MISSING

ROBERT C. SHALER

FREE PRESS
NEW YORK LONDON TORONTO SYDNEY

TO THE FAMILIES WHO LOST THEIR LOVED ONES

*f*P

FREE PRESS
A Division of Simon & Schuster, Inc.
1230 Avenue of the Americas
New York, NY 10020

FREE PRESS and colophon are trademarks
of Simon & Schuster, Inc.

For information regarding special discounts for bulk purchases,
please contact Simon & Schuster Special Sales at 1-800-456-6798
or business@simonandschuster.com

Designed by ISPN Publishing

Manufactured in the United States of America

10 9 8 7 6 5 4 3 2 1

Library of Congress Cataloging-in-Publication Data is available.

ISBN-13: 978-0-7432-7520-0
ISBN-10:   0-7432-7520-9

CONTENTS

PART II MORE THAN SCIENCE

PART III WINDING DOWN AND MOVING ON

PREFACE

New York City has been host to a number of the nation's historic mass-fatality events, some of which have led to new legislation or to sweeping social change. In 1904, the steamer the *General Slocum* was making its annual three-hour excursion from the pier at East Third Street to Long Island. At the Hell Gate, a turbulent and treacherous part of the East River, the steamer caught fire and sank, officially killing 1,021 and perhaps as many bodies were never recovered. David Von Drehle's *Triangle: The Fire That Changed America* tells the story of the Triangle Shirtwaist Company fire of 1911, which killed 146 people, 123 of whom were women. That tragedy was an eerie prophecy of the World Trade Center attacks on September 11, 2001, because many jumped to their deaths to avoid being burned.

The Triangle fire changed the sweatshop practices of unscrupulous employers, and the *General Slocum* disaster motivated federal and state regulators to improve the emergency equipment on passenger ships. After the World Trade Center attacks, we witnessed the formation of the Department of Homeland Security and our nation's formal declaration of war against terrorism.

This book, however, is not about social change or legislation or even the events of September 11 that changed the course of our nation and its attitude about terrorism. It's about people and identifying the victims of a mass-fatality event, specifically those who perished in the World Trade Center towers. It is not about the heroic work of the Armed Forces DNA Identification Laboratory, which identified those who died that day in the plane that crashed in Shanksville, Pennsylvania, or the one that slammed into the Pentagon. It's about allowing families to move on. Mostly, though, it is the story of un-named men and women who toiled on behalf of those families.

Identifying bodies from mass fatalities in the early twentieth cen-tury involved much less precision than it does now. Identifying those lost on the *General Slocum* was a harrowing experience for relatives who searched through charred remains at the morgue to find their loved ones. Finding loved ones after the Triangle Shirtwaist Com-pany fire was no less harsh. Families had to parade past burned and disfigured bodies lying in caskets and attempt to locate their loved ones based almost solely on recognizing familiar physical features, clothing, or jewelry. Today, identifying our loved ones is mostly a sci-entific endeavor, employing medicine, dentistry, and DNA. It is hoped that our modern practices render the experience less ghoulish from that which families endured in the past.

Traditionally, DNA has played a minor to moderate role in the process. In commercial airliner crashes, a manifest of the passengers exists, and the recovered bodies, though many are badly fragmented, are mostly intact. Dental records, fingerprints, and personal effects often suffice to make the majority of the identifications. Routine DNA testing, the kind that all American forensic DNA laboratories perform daily, is mostly used for reassociating fragments to the re-mains of someone already identified or for identifying remains when other methods fail.

The World Trade Center was different. Larger in scope and oc-curring in two towering public office buildings that also housed a mass-transit hub, the World Trade Center had no official manifest to tell us who or how many were missing. In fact, it took more than two years to obtain a working manifest. There may still be names missing from the list, because we know undocumented immigrants worked there as well.

The falling buildings fragmented everything in their wake, most especially the people. The recovery process was prolonged—nearly nine months—and the World Trade Center rubble burned at near or higher than cremation temperatures for three months, accelerating the decomposition of the remains and affecting the quality of the DNA. Possibly, too, many were entirely cremated and will never be identified. Dental and fingerprint records certainly could not suffice, thrusting DNA into a prominent role in identifying the missing. Sadly, we will never identify everyone who perished. Many were likely cremated from either being in close proximity to or in the rubble that burned for three months, or if they had been in the fireball when the planes exploded. As of April 2005, when the process was suspended, we had identified only 1,592 out of the presumed 2,749 who died.

When asked if I would share my personal account of the DNA effort to identify the missing in the aftermath of the World Trade Center disaster, my first impulse was to say no. My emotions had been intensely private, something I was not ready to share. On reflection, however, I realized that the DNA effort, though mentioned frequently in the print and broadcast media, remained mysterious to most. Telling a family that "DNA made the identification" grossly oversimplified the extent and complexity of the work.

I also realized that many of my staff as well as others at the Office of Chief Medical Examiner (OCME) had chosen to dedicate their lives to this work so that families who lost loved ones might find closure. Since this has been the largest and most scrutinized forensic investigation in United States history, I believe it is important to document for the historical record the heroic efforts of those who were an integral part of the DNA effort.

The purpose of this book is to show for the first time the behind-the-scenes activity of the World Trade Center DNA identification effort. Also, this account is about integrity and how New York City's OCME staff, under the guidance of Dr. Charles Hirsch, refused to hide its mistakes. While this book is about the people who made the World Trade Center identifications, it is also about science. I apologize if some of the text seems esoteric, but I believe it is important to include the science so that readers can understand the complexity of what we faced.

Throughout the World Trade Center DNA identification effort, the print and broadcast media credited me with having conceived, orchestrated, and directed the DNA effort. While that's mostly true, many contributed their expertise, thoughts, and time. These folks are absent from the official record. They deserve credit for their contributions, and I firmly believe Americans need to know who they are and the roles they played.

Still, this is my account of the DNA effort that began on September 11 and continued for more than three years, long after the rest of the working world had moved on. It records the facts as I remember them. If these disagree with others' accounts of the specific sequence of events, then I apologize for the failures of my memory.

What this book will not do is point a finger. It is not meant to be an exposé. Not that there haven't been mistakes, errors in judgment, and personal conflicts. There have. What's important, though, is that given the chaos and the ensuing emotionally exhausting work, everyone associated with the DNA effort worked to the very best of their ability, most going well beyond what would reasonably be expected.

I suppose I was lucky. When Tuesday, September 11, 2001, dawned and most of the world witnessed the attacks on the World Trade Center, I naïvely underestimated the magnitude of the task facing me. I never stopped to consider how long the project would take, the effect it would have on my life and family, or especially the emotional toll it would exact.

Thankfully, there has been a silver lining: the families who lost their loved ones. These wonderful people bonded with me and my staff, made us feel wanted and important, consoled us, and showed us why our efforts were worthwhile. Too often, I'm afraid, we agonized over our work and worried about the effect it was having on these families, eschewing the emotional toll it was taking on us. We often cried at our computers and at weekly meetings with the families. Sometimes we high-fived after identifying someone or we'd steal away to an out-of-the-way corner to be alone or simply go for a walk to deal with our emotions. And we hugged.

By February 2005 we had taken the technology as far as it could go and announced that the work would end, for now, although it took until April before the entire staff had actually paused and a letter had been sent to the families. Officially, the OCME was pausing with the hope and expectation that future technology would allow others to reanalyze those remains that still held some DNA. Even before the announcement, I had decided that, when we finished this phase of the work, I would retire. After twenty-five years at the medical examiner's office, I doubted anything could be as important in my career as identifying those who died on September 11, 2001. The families and the community honored me, and for that, I am humbled and will be eternally grateful. Mostly, I want to thank my colleagues who stayed the course. Without them, hundreds of families would never have had their loved ones returned. They were the real heroes of the World Trade Center DNA work. And for them, I have the highest regard and admiration. They are simply the best, ever.

Robert C. Shaler
August 1, 2005

PART I
CHAOS AND UNCERTAINTY

1   SEPTEMBER 11, 2001

I directed the Forensic Biology Department, also known as the DNA lab, at New York City's Office of Chief Medical Examiner (OCME), which routinely analyzes biological evidence in more than three thousand criminal cases annually. The vast majority of these are sexual assaults and homicides. The laboratory is the largest public forensic DNA laboratory in the United States. Although it was housed at the OCME, newspapers erroneously referred to it as the New York City Police Department's DNA laboratory. Even the mayor's office had it confused, when as recently as April 2005, it made public statements suggesting that the DNA laboratory was part of the police department.

The laboratory is located in the OCME penthouse, the sixth floor of the agency's headquarters building, and occupies approximately 12,000 square feet. The laboratory turned out an annual average of more than 1,200 DNA profiles in homicides and sexual assault cases. On September 11, 2001, I was managing 105 people, most of whom were young scientists in the early stages of their careers. Years earlier, after a particularly raucous Christmas party, other OCME staffers had dubbed us the "young and the restless." It fit. I love New York, but I lived in New Jersey, which meant I had to endure a 63-mile commute each way. I hated commuter traffic, so I tailored my travel to arrive at work around 5:30 A.M. and then spent the first hour or so catching up and responding to e-mails. Then I would dive into the boxes of cases that lined the wall of my small office, reviewing them and entering statistics into a database, which is what I was doing on that sunny Tuesday morning when the fire alarm went off at about 7:30 A.M.

The alarm had the bothersome habit of going off when there really wasn't a problem, so I did what I always did: I ignored it. I was certain someone would exclaim "false alarm" over the speaker system. That was SOP, standard operating procedure. So I tuned out the incessant, irritating bell and siren and continued working. Seconds later, I heard a loud, persistent pounding on the lab door. The noise was so loud that it forced me out of my chair and to the door, where I found firefighters gesturing madly at the door, demanding I open it.

A word of caution: if you value your doors, do what firefighters want. They'd rather break down a door than succumb to the more mundane solution—using a key—especially if the key isn't readily available. They have a job to do and nothing stands in the way of their getting it done. For firefighters, time is a precious commodity, which they dare not waste on false alarms.

Unfortunately for the New York City Fire Department, the OCME building seemed to know this and had been toying with them for years. One would think these macho professionals would have known its peculiarities by this time, because the building's ghosts apparently delighted in vexing them with false alarms. Maybe that's why the door was still intact when I greeted them.

That Tuesday's early-morning goblin was the smoke detector located in a storage room at the rear of the DNA lab. This detector had a habit of creating problems, usually during regular working hours, though it rarely rousted New York's Bravest. For some reason, this single smoke detector was sensitive to almost anything: dust, poltergeists, or things cosmic. I learned later that dust left over from the lab's renovation project years earlier had gotten inside it and it had never been cleaned.

The firefighters bulled past me, demanding I show them the culprit room. Ever the dutiful civil servant, I escorted them to the back of the lab, pointed to the door, and watched. They attempted to open the door but found it locked.

"Who has the key?" one firefighter asked gruffly.

"I might have one in my office. I'm not sure whether it'll work,"

I said, knowing it didn't but hoping to stall them until I could find Nick Fusco, our building facilities supervisor, before they invoked their city-given right to splinter the door. I glanced over my shoulder as I left in time to see one firefighter feeling the perimeter of the door for heat.

I reached Nick on the Nextel radio, and he radioed the evidence custodian, who was supposed to have a key, but didn't. Then Nick instructed me to go to his office, where he said there should be a set of keys lying on his desk. After about twenty minutes, I returned to the lab, fully expecting to find an open storage room and door shards strewn across the corridor. Instead, I found only one firefighter, who made a cursory inspection for fire-like signs after I opened the door, then left quickly; too quickly, I thought. I had never seen the FDNY so passive, which I thought was strange and out of character even though it was a common false alarm. I had no way of knowing this was the prelude to a very strange day.

My managerial staff and I had set aside Tuesday mornings to meet. We started at 8:30 and usually finished sometime after 10:00. The meetings gave us a chance to get ourselves on the same page, sort out the week's problems, address pending issues, and establish lab policy. Dr. Howard Baum, my deputy director, and Dr. Mecki Prinz, Marie Samples, Dr. Pasquale Buffolino, and Karen Dooling (the latter two left the OCME in December 2001) were my assistant directors. We were in the midst of what I'm certain was an important discussion when at about 8:50, someone knocked on the conference room door.

Ralph Ristenbatt, my MESATT (Medical Examiner's Scientific Assessment and Training Team) supervisor, stood there, clearly agitated and gesturing for me to join him in the hall. Ralph was not in the habit of interrupting our weekly meeting, so I excused myself and left the room, shutting the door behind me.

An experienced forensic scientist and crime reconstruction expert, Ralph was in his midthirties. He had been at the OCME for more than ten years and was still enthusiastic about his work.

I was expecting a heads-up about MESATT. On autopilot, my mind was already hearing something like "Detective Such-and-Such wants us to examine the blood spatter at a scene in the Bronx."

"What's up?" I said.

"A plane just hit the World Trade Center."

"What?" I said, not certain I heard him correctly.

"A plane—"

"What kind?"

"Don't know. Just happened—small—twin-engine Cessna or something like that."

"Bodies?"

Ralph shook his head. "Don't know."

"How much damage?"

He shrugged. "I don't know."

My mind was reeling, screaming, "It's a mistake. This didn't happen. Who is that fucking stupid?" I poked my head back into the conference room.

"A plane just hit the World Trade Center."

Astonishment and disbelief do not adequately describe the expressions on the faces of my management staff.

"How big was it?" someone asked, a female voice.

Ralph said, "It's a small plane. Schomburg wants MESATT to help set up a temporary morgue at the World Trade Center ASAP. We have to get going."

I hesitated. If Dave Schomburg, the OCME director of medico-legal investigations, was setting up a temporary morgue, there had to be bodies. "Sure," I said, still stunned. "Get going."

My mind leaped into hyperdrive, flooding me with questions: How many bodies? When would they be coming to the OCME?

I followed Ralph to the elevator. I needed to see my boss, Dr. Charles Hirsch, the chief medical examiner, and Dave Schomburg, whom I found in the lobby. His face appeared taut, his expression intense. He quickly told me that two major airliners had hit the buildings, one pounding into each building with passengers aboard, and there was a fire.

My mind was having trouble comprehending the enormity of what I had heard. There would be bodies, hundreds if the planes were full. Thousands if the buildings were filled with workers.

By now, I was on First Avenue in front of the OCME building with Chuck Hirsch, Dave Schomburg, Dan Stevelman, the director of facilities maintenance, Ralph, and the rest of the MESATT team.

In his midsixties, Chuck Hirsch was unquestionably the most rational and stable person I'd met in my life. Always well tailored, he always seemed in control of himself and his surroundings, someone whose clothes perfectly fit his lithe, athletic body. He had become my role model. Chuck's exemplary career had taken him from Ohio, where he trained, to Suffolk County, New York, where he had been the chief medical examiner, and finally to New York City. In his tenure as chief medical examiner of this country's largest medical examiner's office, he reinvented an office mired in turmoil and scandal and turned it into a pillar of efficiency and professionalism, recognized everywhere as a world-class operation.

"How many dead?" I asked Chuck.

"We don't know," he replied, his usually calm demeanor now clearly fragile.

"The DNA lab will be ready," I said with more conviction than I felt.

Chuck barely glanced at me. He simply nodded, then turned and strode to his car with Dianne Christie, a medicolegal investigator, in tow. Ralph was standing on the running board of a white OCME Ford Excursion, the MESATT vehicle. The other members of MESATT—supervising criminalists Brian Gestring and Mark Desire (criminalists are scientists who specialize in the scientific analysis of evidence) and OCME resident forensic anthropologist Amy Mundorff (forensic anthropologists are experts who study bones in order to identify the individual; they can also help pathologists determine the cause and manner of death)—were climbing inside. Dan Stevelman left too, but I don't remember seeing him get into a vehicle.

I was of two minds. I desperately wanted to be a part of what was happening downtown, to witness it firsthand. I started walking toward Ralph but changed my mind. My responsibility was to prepare the lab. Ralph and MESATT would be okay. It was the first real decision I made that Tuesday. For me, it was a lucky one.

I hadn't seen the planes hit the Twin Towers either on TV or in person, as millions had. But I had the gut feeling that DNA might become important. On my way back to the sixth-floor DNA conference room, I listened to a radio broadcast. Although I knew it intellectually, my mind stubbornly refused to accept that the World Trade Center had been attacked again. I thought back to 1993, when terrorists had set off a bomb in the parking garage beneath the complex, murdering six people. The bastards had returned to finish the job.

In the conference room, my assistant directors were already working to reorganize the laboratory. We needed to establish teams to accept remains into the laboratory, track them, extract the DNA, and then analyze it. Remains would start coming in later that day and we had to be ready.

The Department of Forensic Biology had a staff of 105 scientists. A lack of space in the OCME building forced us to split up. We occupied the entire sixth floor of the OCME building at 520 First Avenue, the corner of 30th Street and First Avenue (eventually, the World Trade Center DNA identification unit would occupy part of a room on the second floor), and we had a satellite site on part of the fourth floor of the administration building at Bellevue Hospital, four blocks away. The Bellevue lab was a makeshift facility where criminalists examined biological evidence from criminal investigations occurring in the city. Cuttings removed from the evidence came to the sixth floor in the OCME building, where other criminalists analyzed the DNA. We had a modern facility in the planning stages, a thirteen-story, 300,000-plus-square-foot building devoted to forensic biology that would consolidate the laboratory under one roof, but it was years from completion.

While conferring with my managerial staff, I was having trouble concentrating. This might seem strange given the daunting task facing us, but my mind wandered. I kept thinking about a presentation given a couple of years earlier by Dr. Ron Forney of the Royal Canadian Mounted Police to the New York State DNA Subcommittee. He had outlined how the RMCP had used DNA to identify the missing after Swissair Flight 111 crashed off the coast of Nova Scotia in September 1998 and 229 lost their lives. The Canadians had analyzed more than 1,200 samples using an approach that was both efficient and logical. I had been impressed. Instead of singling out one laboratory to perform the DNA-typing efforts, they had employed several of the country's public forensic labs, sending samples as far as Vancouver to get the testing done quickly. The DNA data came back to their headquarters facility in Ottawa, where scientists analyzed them. Dr. Benoit Leclair made the identifications using an Excel spreadsheet that he had programmed.

At that time, Dr. Barry Duceman, director of the New York State Police Biological Sciences laboratory in Albany, and I often said that New York State needed a software package like Benoit's. We both thought we should either obtain a copy of Benoit's program or develop one. It was an idea that never materialized. Chuck Hirsch and I had several short conversations on the subject over the years. Separately, we urged New York State to develop a DNA implementation plan for mass disasters. Mark Dale, inspector of the New York State Forensic Investigation Center at the time and Barry Duceman's boss, also agreed. The only movement toward this end came after Chuck contacted the state, which resulted in Ron Forney's presentation. Then nothing happened. Mass-disaster preparation, everyone agreed, was important—what self-respecting politician would disagree?—but the short-term, more politically expedient issues always took precedence. Mass disasters had clearly been relegated to everyone's back burner.

While one part of my mind listened to my managerial staff attempt to deal with the emerging situation, another part lamented not having Benoit's software. I guessed the Armed Forces DNA Identification Laboratory had a version and I wondered whether the FBI had something. Without the appropriate software to help make the identifications, we were hopelessly lost.

I realized that I was of little help to my staff, who were doing a stellar job of reorganizing the lab. Although I certainly wanted to be a part of their discussion, I decided to see how the OCME as an agency had been organized, which certainly would have a critical effect on the laboratory. How would bodies get into the OCME? How would specimens come to the laboratory? Which samples would the medical examiners collect? What about chain of custody? Would it be tight and foolproof? What about sample mixups? That thought scared the crap out of me.

I left the conference room and was heading out of the lab to find Dave Schomburg when my cell phone vibrated.

"Bob, you won't fucking believe this!" Ralph screamed. "People are hanging out of the building. Oh fuck! Someone jumped. People are fucking jumping! This is horrible!"

"Jesus Christ," was all that I could muster. "Are you all right?"

Visions of people falling 110 stories filled my brain. I couldn't talk.

"This is unbelievable."

"Where are you?"

"In front of the Marriott. Jesus Christ. This is fucking horrible," he cried. "Bob, you won't believe what it's like, the sound—when they hit."

Today, when I see photos or videos of people jumping from the buildings, I still hear the horror in his voice.

I instructed him to stay in touch and to be careful. I returned to the conference room.

Then the South Tower fell. It was 10:02.

Shocked, we ran into the lab and listened to the broadcast. None of us could believe what had happened. Then the North Tower fell at 10:29. I went to my office and tried calling my wife, Fran, but I couldn't get an outside line. Frustrated, I went downstairs to the lobby, where Dave Schomburg grabbed my arm and pulled me aside. "We've lost contact with Dr. Hirsch and MESATT," he said.

I just stared at him. My heart sank. I fought back tears and prayed silently. With a heavy heart, I returned to my office. Howard Baum, Marie Samples, and Karen Dooling were just leaving the conference room. "Schomburg told me Dan Stevelman's on his way to the hospital," I said.

"How bad?" Howie asked.

"I don't know." I was having trouble finding the words. "And we've lost communication with Dr. Hirsch and MESATT."

Karen was standing in the doorway to Mecki Prinz's office. Tears welled up in her eyes.

Tears flooded mine. "We don't know anything for certain, yet," I managed to say.

I couldn't just stand there. I felt like I had to be doing something, anything. The lab was in good hands, so I returned to the lobby. The remainder of the morning seemed like a blur. I found myself running between my managerial staff, checking on how the lab setup was progressing, and the lobby, where I was gathering information on the number of people who had died.

By midafternoon, Dave Schomburg, Shiya Ribowsky, the deputy director for medicolegal investigations, and Dr. Mark Flomenbaum, deputy chief medical examiner, had gathered the entire OCME staff into a group. They were about to explain the body-handling procedures and what was expected of them when I walked into the lobby.

I was surprised that no one thought to include the DNA laboratory. Maybe they believed that DNA would not become a critical part of the identification process. Perhaps it was simply an oversight, given the craziness of that day. The autopsies would be done by medical examiners who, historically, thought in terms of teeth, fingerprints, and body X-rays for identifying remains. These are the most widely employed techniques for identifying remains in mass disasters, and DNA had not been used to any great extent in mass-fatality events. Did they know about how critical the DNA work had been in the Swissair crash? When TWA Flight 800 crashed off the coast of Long Island in 1998, the medical examiner had decided that DNA would not be important and had to go back to families after they had remains in order to return pieces that had been identified using DNA. Instead of getting angry, I chalked up the oversight to someone's assumption that if the DNA laboratory was needed, it would be a simple matter to send the samples to the lab, as though something like this occurred every day.

I was learning a difficult lesson. Scientists have never been included in mass-disaster drills because preparedness planning typically focused on containment, rescue, and recovery operations. Identifying remains was never on the preparedness radar, which meant scientists and medical examiners would always be secondary responders, performing a perceived secondary role. This is true only in the sense that this role happens second. It is no less important. Both first and secondary responders are necessary and both should be part of the preparation effort. In the instance of the World Trade Center attacks, first responders worked tirelessly for nine months. In contrast, my staff would work doggedly for more than three years.

So, if I had questions about what the lab's role would be, why didn't the others? Did they know which samples to collect or how much? What if the remains were decomposed or charred? It did not matter how many drills one had attended, no one had been through anything like this. Unlike those in charge of investigations, no one in the DNA lab, me included, had been invited to attend the semi-annual mass-disaster drills held in the city. Interestingly, the administrative staff of the OCME still attends these drills. DNA still does not. Other than receiving samples to analyze, I was at a loss to understand what those who were running the show expected. How were we supposed to interact with the medical staff? I needed guidelines, and from what I saw, there were none.

I gently pushed my way into the crowd of OCME staffers and listened to Shiya and Dave outline their plan. Simply hearing what they had to say alleviated some of my anxiety, though not all. The good news was that they had what sounded like a well-thought-out, logical plan. The bad news was that they failed to mention the DNA laboratory. That worried me considerably.

I yanked Shiya aside and asked him to explain how he planned to obtain samples and get them to the lab. He assured me that everything was in place. I have a great deal of respect for Shiya, but I was still not convinced. I needed to see exactly how the process would work.

I'm not sure whether Shiya recognized my concern or just wanted to placate me, but he escorted a small group to the basement, where the morgue is located, and explained his vision for how bodies would be accessioned and how the examination in the morgue area was to proceed. ("Accessioning" refers to the acceptance of remains—actually any evidence—into the OCME or the DNA laboratory. This is a process referred to as the chain of custody, which is the legal record that documents when evidence was brought to the laboratory or OCME, where it was stored, when it left, and who handled it. Basically, it is a legal history of the evidence handling.)

He explained how we would track cases, how remains would move from the dropoff area on 30th Street, to the autopsy area, and then through dental X-ray, body X-ray, and fingerprints, and then back to 30th Street, where they would be stored in refrigerated trailers because there would not be sufficient room in the OCME coolers.

The OCME procurement group supervised by Lorraine Kelly obtained the first two trailers, high cubes, that arrived that day. The one from a local fish company was designated to hold the remains of members of the services—firefighters, policemen, and other uniformed personnel—and the other was for civilian remains. Refrigerated tractor trailers from UPS, Ben & Jerry's, and other companies began arriving on 9/12. Shiya segregated them on 30th Street into preprocessing and postprocessing stations; "processing" refers to the autopsy. At one point, tractor trailers formed a line on Second Avenue from 30th Street to 38th Street. Eventually, they lined both sides of 30th Street between First Avenue and the FDR Drive. Dave

Schomburg suggested putting the trailers in a vacant area at the end of 30th Street between 29th and 30th Streets behind the old Bellevue psychiatric hospital. The Department of Transportation paved the area and the sixteen tractor trailers were lined up, eight on a side, their back ends facing each other. Eventually, on October 11, the trailers were covered by a large white tent. Before that, Lorraine Kelly arranged for a party tarp to cover the remains, protect workers from the elements, and keep prying cameras from photographing the remains. The area at the FDR end of 30th Street became known as Memorial Park, a resting place for the remains until a memorial is built at the WTC site.

Each recovered remain—no longer referred to as "bodies"—would receive a DM01 number, which stood for "Disaster Manhattan 2001." Over the next several days, I learned that a remain could be anything from a mostly intact body to a foot, a finger, a single piece of bone or flesh, a tooth, or even a single hair. Sometimes a DM number would be assigned to something like a piece of plastic that was covered by a light gray dust. The dust resulted from the huge gray cloud that erupted over downtown when the buildings fell. It was ubiquitous, so that visually distinguishing between pieces of plastic and bone fragments was extremely difficult, if not impossible.

When I happened on the meeting in the lobby, I thought it had been called by Dave and Shiya and was upset because no one had alerted me. Years later, I learned that Shiya, too, had happened onto the meeting much like I did. Typically, however, he had carved his own role and did most of the talking, which led me to believe that he had been an organizer. In fact, no one had invited him either, yet he was responsible for World Trade Center investigations, confirming the identifications and notifying the families.

That Tuesday was not the first time we had reorganized the laboratory. I had asked my staff to reorganize the lab in 1996. At that time, I needed to find a way to alleviate a huge backlog of cases and reduce an obscene case-turnaround time, which had grown to greater than one hundred days. A typical approach for solving these problems is to increase the staff. However, before I felt comfortable asking the city for more staff and resources, I believed we had to streamline the lab processes and become as efficient as possible using existing resources. If I could demonstrate to the city's Office of Management and Budget, the bean counters, that we had done everything possible to make the lab efficient using existing staff and equipment and still could not lower the backlog or turnaround time significantly, I would be in a stronger position to ask for more, especially given how important DNA was becoming to the criminal justice system.

I challenged my management staff to do more with less, and asked them to think out of the box and reinvent how a forensic lab does business. The existing forensic laboratory paradigm had become archaic, especially for a large laboratory: one analyst, one case, one workup, one report, one testimony. In this scenario, a single analyst works a case from beginning to end: examining the evidence, cutting out a bloodstain and/or other stains, performing the DNA testing, writing the report, and finally testifying in court. I wanted the laboratory to adopt more of a clinical model, which meant analyzing samples in batches instead of one at a time.

Over several weeks, we developed what we called the rotation system, where the staff were assigned weekly to an analytical station, a rotation. The beauty of the system was its flexibility. It was easy to reorganize the lab to accommodate specific needs, such as rush cases and other emergencies, by simply adding a new rotation to the schedule and assigning staff and someone to supervise that new rotation.

By day's end on September 11 the disaster rotations had been put into place. We identified the staff to work them, suspended regular casework for the foreseeable future, and considered canceling staff vacations, which we did weeks later but for only a limited time. Lydia DeCastro, a supervising criminalist, assumed the important responsibility of supervising one of these new rotations that would accession remains, extract the DNA from tissues, and send samples to vendor laboratories.

A scientist in her midthirties and about five feet four, Lydia has a strong work ethic. I had first met her twelve years earlier when she worked in my laboratory as a summer intern. After rotating through the OCME working in various sections, she decided forensic biology fit her career aspirations, although, at the time, she was trapped in the OCME toxicology laboratory, where she had to labor for four years before I had an opening. Before the World Trade Center attacks, she had been working on her master's degree part-time at John Jay College of Criminal Justice and was an accomplished forensic DNA scientist.

Lydia is a no-nonsense lady who rarely hesitated to put me in my place when I did something stupid, like not keep her in the loop for information she needed for her group. I believed she was the perfect choice, and she seemed delighted to accept the critical task of tracking disaster samples. We staffed her rotation with some of the lab's newest members, a group of eager young professionals, many of whom had started their forensic careers on September 10. When I saw them in the laboratory working on the remains, I wondered whether they had the stomach to stick it out.

Most of them did, and I must say, I've never been more proud of a group of young people. They began their forensic biology careers under the best and the worst of circumstances. It was the best because working on the World Trade Center project may well have been the most important assignment of their careers. It was the worst because I could not have imagined a more gruesome task for young professionals on their first forensic job. Sometimes I thought it was a shame that their careers began like that, with little hope of working on anything else that important. I'm the lucky one because my OCME career ended with the World Trade Center work.

We lacked the tools Lydia needed to do the job properly or efficiently: no bar-coding capability, no laboratory information management system, or LIMS, to keep track of samples. LIMS are software systems designed to streamline laboratory processes by eliminating manual chores. These can be simple evidence-tracking systems, which is how we initially used the BEAST (Bar Coded Evidence Analysis Statistics and Tracking, a LIMS program developed by Porter Lee Corporation). These systems vary widely, depending on the application. They can become extremely complex when programmed to interface instruments, schedule work, prepare reports, develop management statistics, and track samples using bar codes.

When remains first arrived at the lab, Lydia's group had to track them manually, which was an ominous and daunting task. I thought it was nearly an impossible job to do error free, and I had the sinking feeling that we would mix up samples and return the wrong body to a family. The process had nightmare written all over it.

Still, we had an advantage over most American forensic laboratories. We were the largest public forensic DNA lab in the country and had been processing cases, tracking samples, and performing thousands of DNA tests manually without mixups. But we were asking for problems if we had to track a year's worth of work or more monthly. Fatigue would settle in and we would make mistakes.

Marie Samples and Lydia went to Staples and bought logbooks. Then they instructed the clerical and lab staff how to prepare manila folders—that was how we tracked routine criminal cases, which was the only way we could do it.

Each manila folder had a unique, sequential forensic biology case number (e.g., FB01–D0001), where each file was for one of the remains, as yet unnamed. FB stood for forensic biology and 01 the year. The D differentiated World Trade Center cases from regular criminal casework and stood for disaster. The core sequential number was designed to match the core DM number that the medical examiner assigned to the remains as they were autopsied. Each remain had a bar-code label, which Lydia's group unfortunately could not yet read.

Originally, we chose to extract the DNA and produce DNA profiles by testing for short tandem repeats, or STRs, in-house. STRs are biological markers that are inherited from our parents and vary widely among people. Testing for an STR at each of thirteen different regions of the DNA results in a virtually unique DNA profile, referred

to as an STR profile. STRs in identical twins are the same. STR testing is the foundation of forensic DNA testing worldwide. Even before we received samples, I was thinking about getting the analysis
started. I was also interested in the quality of the samples as they
came into the lab. Lisa Palumbo Desire, a supervising criminalist and
Mark Desire's wife, accepted the disaster STR rotation. This meant
her group would produce the DNA profiles we needed for making
identifications.

By late that afternoon, we had reorganized the lab. Albeit with
some trepidation, I thought we were as ready as we could ever be. File
folders were in place, supervisors had been assigned, and scientists
had been identified to work the disaster rotations. Although we had
little information from the World Trade Center site, except for what
was being reported in the media, for the first time that day, I was beginning to relax somewhat.

Working a mass disaster was something I never asked for or
wanted, though I had always expected that working in a forensic laboratory in New York City meant my turn would come. It was a given,
only a matter of time. I assumed it would be an airliner crash or a
bombing. Once, I mentioned to Marie Samples and Howard Baum
that my worst-case scenario would be an airplane crashing into a
building. I hadn't conceived of two planes and two buildings. And
certainly not the Twin Towers. Actually, my vision included the Em-
pire State Building.

Earlier in the day, I suggested to Mark Flomenbaum, who was responsible for scheduling the medical examiners for World Trade Center autopsy duty, that a DNA scientist should work with the medical
examiners to select appropriate specimens for DNA analysis. My
thought was to head off or minimize future problems. Mark apparently mentioned this to Shiya, who agreed and took my suggestion a
step further. He agreed that a DNA scientist should be in the morgue
to answer questions, but expanded the plan to having a DNA person
present at each autopsy table, on a 24/7 basis.

That first night, we had only a handful of DNA lab staff to work
in the autopsy area. Our official morgue schedule did not begin until

the next day. Howard Baum and I stayed along with my other assistant directors Marie and Mecki. Others included Theresa Caragine, Brett Hutchinson, and Chris Kamnik. Radio broadcasts had been announcing that the bridges and tunnels to New Jersey were closed, so I probably could not have gone home even if I had wanted to. Many months later, I remember seeing a documentary on September 11 that showed a sign on the New Jersey Turnpike that read "New York City Closed."

The reality was that it didn't matter. I was not about to leave. My anguish and anger at what had happened ran too deeply. I felt compelled to stay, to help, to be available, to do whatever I could.

Inside me, too, was the ever-present objective, detached side— the forensic scientist who needed to see what the devastation had done to those who died inside the buildings. It wasn't a morbid curiosity, but more a need to fill an information gap. I have had the unfortunate privilege to have worked with dead bodies for more than thirty years, many decomposing and mutilated, many disfigured and twisted from automobile crashes, burned from fires, or bloated after floating in the Hudson River. But I'd never seen bodies from a mass disaster.

I had seen photos and listened to the descriptions from my colleagues who had worked on airliner crashes. These images had been popping in and out of my mind all day, and I was curious to know how they would compare to those who had died that day.

By 5:00 P.M. I was exhausted, but a nervous energy lurking just below the surface kept my energy levels high. I was hungry, too. Someone suggested that several of us catch a bite to eat, so we trudged to Mumbles on Third Avenue and ordered dinner. We had been there only a few minutes when, around 6:00 P.M., Mark Flomenbaum called.

"The first bodies will be here in about thirty minutes," he said, simultaneously excited yet somber.

I took a deep breath and looked at Howard Baum. "They want us in the morgue."

Butterflies quickly invaded my stomach. I now realized my life had changed forever. Howard and I left the restaurant and headed back to the OCME without having eaten. We asked if someone would bring our sandwiches back to the lab. I have a vague recollection of sitting in my office, alone, thoroughly exhausted and eating in the wee hours of the morning.

We returned to the lab, put on our lab coats, and went to the triage area in the morgue, where we slipped on goggles and latex gloves. About 7:30, the first remains arrived in EMS trucks. The first body was that of a firefighter. A short ceremony on 30th Street led by firefighters emphasized the solemn moment and gave us time to pay our respects and steel our nerves. I don't remember seeing a dry eye in the morgue.

The gruesome process of identifying those unfortunate people had begun. I was uncharacteristically nervous and consciously had to prepare myself for whatever was about to happen. The waiting, with its attendant anticipation, had created an intense anxiety, and I found myself pacing in the morgue. Then, more remains arrived in trucks, and morgue attendants started unloading body bag after body bag, placing each onto a stainless steel autopsy tray. I took a deep breath and walked to an autopsy. I chose to work with medical examiner Dr. Stephanie Fiore.

My breathing came in rapid spurts as a morgue attendant unzipped the first body bag. I swallowed hard. A wave of nausea washed through me and I struggled to fight back tears as I got my first glimpse of what would become an interminable parade of human destruction.

My time in the autopsy area would diminish over the next several days, though I went there daily. My scientific side had to keep pace with the changing quality of the remains, as tissue inevitably decomposes over time. There was a personal side, too: a burning need to be close to the medical examiners and all the other professionals who were working hard to make sense out of chaos. That personal side also needed to be close to those who lost their lives.

That first night many of the remains seemed to be fairly intact, though fragmented, disfigured, and burned, most badly. Many had been crushed from falling pieces of the buildings. And there were fragments that I hoped we would eventually reunite with other pieces ripped so violently from that same person. How long would that take? I certainly did not know. From the extensive fragmentation I saw, I knew this: without DNA, those pieces could never be linked together.

2   WHY ME?

Over the years, I've learned that I'm neither the brightest star in the sky nor the dullest. But when I first climbed the steps to the Office of Chief Medical Examiner on November 13, 1978, at thirty-six years old, it didn't matter. I was the new head of the Serology Laboratory (as the Forensic Biology Lab was then known) and I had the enthusiasm and energy of a kid ready to conquer Gotham. I was nervous but felt confident in my ability and comfortable with my new position. I didn't yet know the obstacles I would encounter from the OCME's criminal justice system partner, the New York City Police Department.

The NYPD's reputation for employing forensic science in the 1970s was laughable; to those on the outside, its leaders were considered clueless or, worse, uncaring. The NYPD crime lab had an especially horrible reputation; its crime scene unit labored short-handed, underfunded, and still photographed scenes in black and white. Even worse, proper forensic techniques did not seem to be a priority. The largest of the city's law enforcement arms believed its crime lab was the cat's meow of forensic science. It was not. Those were the dark days of forensic science in New York.

Prior to that day in November 1978, I had no personal experience with New York, so I was not in a position to judge. I quickly learned that even if that awful reputation was true, New Yorkers could not have cared less what I or any outsider thought. Until you'd proven yourself in New York, your track record did not amount to a hill of beans.

On that first day, however, I was oblivious of all that. I believed I had the plum forensic job in the country; I had arrived in forensic science heaven. If I had doubts, they were securely tucked deep inside the recesses of my mind, not to surface until the next day, when I learned that I had inherited a caseload of two thousand homicides, 60 percent of them backlogged, and a staff of only four, including myself. On my third day, I found myself staring dumbfounded into a room on the fifth floor at the OCME filled eyeball-deep with black plastic bags containing homicide physical evidence. Many had lost their tags and were unmarked. This was one of my evidence rooms. I immediately knew that tracking older cases would be a nightmare. At least the room was locked. A cursory inventory told me that the evidence went back perhaps ten years. Astoundingly, there was no obvious cataloging system. I later learned that I had also inherited an almost identical mess on the third floor.

Now I was beginning to worry. What else didn't I know? I had been so anxious to work in New York City that I had made the mistake of accepting only an oral commitment for more staffing, equipment (most of which I had brought with me), and space. Also, there was still the unanswered, nagging question: could I fill my predecessor's famous shoes?

I had met Dr. Alexander Weiner only once and that had been over the telephone. I was working on a Law Enforcement Assistance Administration (forerunner of the National Institute of Justice) research grant while at the University of Pittsburgh and had called Dr. Weiner to ask him about a research problem.

He had said gruffly, "It can't be done. You can't use the system for dried bloodstains." Then he abruptly hung up. Not even a good-bye. I was dumbfounded, but I vowed to prove him wrong. (In the end, we both were right and wrong. I solved the problem, but we never used the system on bloodstains.)

Dr. Weiner was an internationally famous microbiologist. A physician, he was the head of the OCME serology laboratory (employed part-time), had a private medical practice in Brooklyn, and raised rabbits so that he could manufacture his own specialized blood grouping sera (none was available commercially). In the 1930s, his name was synonymous with the discipline of hematology and he was internationally renowned as the codiscoverer of the Rh blood group system. (All mothers know the importance of being either Rh positive or negative.)

I subsequently learned from Dr. Michael Baden, then the chief medical examiner, that Dr. Weiner had been impressed with my work on a Queens, New York, homicide case. While a research forensic scientist at the University of Pittsburgh, I had been contacted by the Queens District Attorney's office asking if I would test some of the evidence. Apparently, Dr. Weiner was impressed by my work and mentioned the work to Dr. Baden. That same year, Dr. Weiner died, and I got the job.

My learning curve at the OCME was steep. Michael had a habit of dragging me into the autopsy room at all hours of the day and night—once so I could see the skullcap of someone who had been given tetracycline as a child. When he shined an ultraviolet light on it, it fluoresced a bright orange. Another time, he called me into the office at 2:00 A.M. so that I could see how someone had dissected his own arm, muscle by muscle, tweezing each out individually and labeling each with a stickpin. It was disgusting and reminded me of my cat anatomy class in college. We went to crime scenes, discussed autopsy results, and argued over how to extract drugs from tissues. It was a terrific learning experience.

In the late 1970s, forensic science wasn't in the public eye like it is today. There were no TV programs like *CSI*, *The New Detectives*, *Cold Case Files*, or *Forensic Files* to woo young scientists into the field, although *Quincy*, starring Jack Klugman, was a popular program. In the 1970s, few science students knew such a career even existed or how to get into it.

I happened into the profession quite accidentally. I received my PhD in biochemistry from Pennsylvania State University and was working as a postdoctoral fellow at the University of Pittsburgh School of

Medicine when I spied an article in the *Pittsburgh Press* touting a series of forensic sleuthing courses being offered by the University of Pittsburgh, Department of Chemistry, and members of the Pittsburgh and Allegheny County Crime Laboratory. The idea of scientific crime detection intrigued me, so I signed up for the courses, which lasted two years. (I did not receive a master's degree in that discipline because I stupidly refused to take a one-credit law class; I already had a master's degree and a PhD.)

I accepted a night job working at the Pittsburgh and Allegheny County Crime Laboratory as a drug chemist and crime scene analyst, although my only hands-on training as a drug chemist came in course work. I had an undergraduate degree in chemistry and my graduate training was in biochemistry, but my real desire was to apply my graduate training to forensic science. I obtained research funding from the Law Enforcement Assistance Administration, which eventually took me to the Aerospace Corporation, where I managed several Law Enforcement Assistance Administration contracts. One resulted in the Bloodstain Analysis System, which could become my edge when I started working at the OCME in 1978. It was the bloodstain analysis standard in the United States for almost a decade.

At that time, most forensic biology (most referred to it as serology) laboratories used isoenzyme genetic markers (inherited biological molecules that vary among people) to individualize semen obtained from sexual assault survivors and bloodstains from crime scenes. There were several of these markers, and usually each was tested individually. Additionally, there were several ways in which to run the test, and this had created a controversy over which was the best. One school of thought was at the University of California in Berkeley and another was at the Metropolitan Police Laboratory in London.

One afternoon in 1976, I received a call from John Sullivan, who was both a friend and the director of the Law Enforcement Assistance Administration's forensic program. He had funds that he had to give to the Aerospace Corporation, but he was concerned because the company had no forensic experience. John was looking for projects. I thought it would be interesting to have a head-to-head competition between the proponents of both systems. I also thought it should be possible to run more than one isoenzyme system at a time. I told John my ideas, which ended up as a statement of work (or SOW), a list of tasks that potential vendors would bid on in order to obtain funding to do the work that would be done by the Aerospace Corporation of El Segundo, California. I was brought in to manage the project, which meant I would have to leave Pittsburgh.

Although the Aerospace Corporation had its headquarters in California, I managed the program from a satellite office in Washington, DC. The projects included research at the University of California at Berkeley, Beckman Instruments in Anaheim, California, and the Aerospace Corporation in El Segundo. The competition was heated and the animosity between the groups became known as the "Starch Wars" (because starch was one of the methods being considered). The end result was the Bloodstain Analysis System that I would take with me to New York.

Early in 1979, my career at the medical examiner's office was in full swing. I was happy and productive, and my learning curve was unabated. Then after almost a year, it changed. Mayor Ed Koch fired Michael Baden and replaced him with Dr. Elliot Gross. It was an ill-fated hiring because Elliot and Michael had always been competitors, both having been trained in forensic pathology by New York's guru medical examiner, Dr. Milton Helpern. The next few years were the darkest of my career.

My relationship with Elliot Gross was strained at best, almost from the beginning. Before he officially started, I had requested an additional scientific position on my staff and had been turned down. I was angry, so I wrote to Manhattan District Attorney Robert Morgenthau, the head of the Department of Health, and others to plead my case, explaining that I would not be responsible for errors if the city refused to support the laboratory. Apparently, my argument fell on sympathetic ears and the position was approved. But when Dr. Gross came on board, he wasn't pleased. Within his first week, he ordered me into his office, accused me of going behind his back, and forbade me from contacting Mr. Morgenthau again.

Our relationship soured further after another incident. I had identified blood on a gun in a homicide case. The district attorney handling the case needed the gun for court. Our records indicated that the gun had been put into the evidence room (the one I had inherited), where it got misplaced among the hundreds of other packages. We searched the room over and over but failed to find it. After a couple of days, the frustrated district attorney called Dr. Gross, who, for some inexplicable reason, contacted the Department of Investigation (DOI). One afternoon, I had returned to my office after testifying in court to find someone sitting at my desk, feet resting on top of it and rummaging through the top drawer. He was a DOI investigator who had been given the task of finding the gun, which I found the next day. Well, my Irish temper exploded. I ordered him out of my office and then charged into Dr. Gross's office and offered him a generous piece of my mind. Whatever relationship we had ceased at that moment.

Dr. Charles Hirsch, the chief medical examiner at the Suffolk County, Long Island, Medical Examiner's Office, asked me to interview to direct his crime lab. I was ecstatic. Chuck Hirsch had a terrific reputation among forensic scientists. He was one of those rare medical examiners who truly appreciated and understood the complementary relationship between forensic medicine and forensic science. I journeyed to what seemed like the end of the earth, almost the easternmost tip of Long Island, and spent the day.

My wife, Fran, and I spent another day looking at real estate. As the day wore on, a sad truth emerged. I would never accept Chuck's offer, though I craved the job. Even if Fran could get a job working in the laboratory there, the cost of living and our budget were in severe conflict. I harbored visions of pushing a shopping cart containing all of my worldly possessions to work each day. Cursing under my breath,

I realized that I would have to remain at the medical examiner's office in New York City under Elliot Gross's control.

The next year, an opportunity came along that I would not pass up. Lifecodes Corporation had developed a forensic DNA test and asked me to develop their forensic business. My job was to introduce forensic DNA testing to the law enforcement community. I accepted and eagerly left the city, vowing never to return.

Once again luck had smiled on me. God had placed me on the ground floor of something novel and groundbreaking. DNA's potential captivated me. In 1987 I left Manhattan for Valhalla, New York, with a renewed vigor. Forensic DNA testing was an emerging field with unprecedented promise.

Unfortunately, life has a way of leveling all playing fields. Eventually, Lifecodes's lure tarnished, and the company that had saved me from forensic science hell in New York under Gross's inept guidance changed presidents. The incoming head of the company did not share my vision, and the company's focus changed. I no longer had my windowed corner office overlooking a sylvan setting in Westchester County. I was banished to the basement, where I shared a windowless storage room with a colleague. My responsibilities diminished and my self-esteem and ego were badly bruised. I was embarrassed and disillusioned.

Then Lady Luck smiled on me once again when Chuck Hirsch reentered my life. In 1989 he replaced Elliot Gross, who had been fired by Mayor Koch, and was given a mandate from the mayor to restore the OCME's reputation, diminished under Dr. Gross's stronghanded management. Part of his plan was to establish a modern forensic DNA laboratory, and he wanted me to accept the challenge.

I certainly wanted it, but my experience with Elliot Gross had soured me on returning to work for the city. I had vowed I would never work for the city again. He asked if I would prepare a plan that he could take to the city's Office of Management and Budget. I agreed. It was my undoing. The city accepted the plan and agreed to fund it, a promise that Chuck used to lure me back. With some trepidation, I agreed. Chuck's challenge to establish a modern forensic molecular biology laboratory was exciting. I needed help and convinced Dr. Howard Baum, a former Lifecodes colleague, to join me.

Howard had gone to Lifecodes's staff after receiving his PhD at Brandeis University five years earlier and made his mark as one of the company's bright molecular biologists. Although Howard and I had significantly different scientific backgrounds, he had always been willing to help me solve problems. With his expertise in molecular biology and mine in forensic science, I thought we had the makings of a great team.

Howard is one of those people whom I affectionately refer to as a "noodge." Sporting a dark beard that later showed some salt, and an off-again, on-again protruding paunch, he often appears tousled, typical of a scientist. He is extremely bright, loves to know everything about most anything—and doesn't hesitate to tell you—and prides himself on his laboratory prowess, although he rarely works in the lab anymore.

Over the years, he made himself into a forensic scientist, learned the rudiments of crime scene processing and investigation, mastered the nuances of the city's civil service system, and learned how to deal with disgruntled, complaining subordinates. He also had a feel for New York City politics.

So, once again my adrenaline and creative juices flowed. Chuck Hirsch's steadfast and singular approach to forensic medicine fascinated me. Now that I was actually working for him, I realized how lucky I was. Like my first boss at Lifecodes, who gave me all the rope I needed to hang myself, Chuck hired people he respected and asked them to do a job. He's a leader whose character and professionalism embody everything I would like to be.

Establishing a world-class scientific facility within the city's procurement system turned into an experience in frustration and uncertainty, subject to the city's political climate and widely swinging budgetary cycles. However, with Chuck Hirsch's unending support, Howard and I did it. Once the laboratory achieved success in solving crimes, aiding NYPD investigations, and putting criminals behind bars, it attracted the attention of the press, which wanted New York stories about how DNA solved crimes.

To be successful, though, Howard and I needed support from both the mayor and law enforcement. In the years before Mayor Rudolph Giuliani, there was precious little. With Chuck's support, I had been submitting proposals to the administration of then-mayor David Dinkins annually, detailing DNA's potential and illustrating how important a tool it would become. I wanted the city to support an expanded DNA laboratory, which because it was part of the OCME, had been tasked to work only homicide cases; I felt they should begin accepting all the sexual assaults in the city. I believed DNA would become the definitive forensic means of identifying rapists.

Our proposals mostly fell on deaf ears, in part, I believe, because the mayor and his staff had been reading about DNA and its reputed unreliability. I'm certain the mayor's staff feared a frenzied media condemnation, especially if some judge threw out the DNA evidence in a celebrated criminal case because he or she did not understand the test—not an uncommon occurrence in those early days of DNA testing. Another reason for not endorsing our proposals was the city's precarious budgetary structure, although funding the DNA laboratory would have barely scraped the surface of its multibillion-dollar budget.

We approached the NYPD for support and managed a meeting with Ray Kelly and his first chief of detectives during Kelly's first term as police commissioner in the early 1990s. After making what I thought was a convincing and logical argument, the chief of detectives said with finality, "DNA don't make no arrests."

The statement not only stung, it embodied the continued and ultimate ignorance of the NYPD's attitude toward forensic science. I was shocked, although admittedly a bit amused. The chief of detectives is someone who is supposed to have his finger on the pulse of all criminal investigations in the city. He should have known the potential value of DNA, which was then frequently chronicled in the press.

Eventually, the lab's success and media attention forced the issue of which agency—the OCME or the New York City Police Department—would control DNA testing for the city's criminal justice system. A high-level meeting in the mid-1990s with Ray Kelly's successor in the police commissioner's office, Howard Safir, the top police brass, then Criminal Justice Coordinator Katie Lapp, and a group from the OCME, including Chuck and me, decided the near-term future of the DNA lab. Importantly, the meeting also decided a more engaging question: which philosophical application of forensic DNA testing would the city endorse? My vision for DNA testing encompassed all crimes in the city. The police department thought more narrowly, considering only sexual assaults and homicides as potential DNA candidates.

After persuasive arguments from both the New York City Police Department and the OCME, it was decided that the DNA lab would stay where it was. I was delighted and relieved.

Magically, it seemed, the funding spigots opened and the lab started growing, doubling its staff every other year. And its impact on the city's criminal justice system was soon clear. By 1998, we began accepting sexual assault cases on a limited basis, with plans to work them all, and it wasn't long before my lab staff was testifying routinely to DNA testing in these cases. Luckily, DNA prevailed. The new administration under former prosecutor Mayor Giuliani understood DNA's importance. By September 2001, we had grown from a staff of four to one hundred five scientists working all of the city's sexual assaults and homicides.

The lab's systematic expansion from 1997 to 2001, on hindsight, seems almost prophetic, as though we had been moving on a collision course with something dramatic. In fact, reflecting on my own professional development, I think some mystical force had been guiding me, preparing me for September 11 and its aftermath.

3 GEARING UP

The transfer of human remains to the lab early on Wednesday, September 12, began slowly and then escalated sharply. By the close of business—closing wasn't really an option—we had 91 specimens, all tissue and blood. On Thursday the number grew to 266 and by Friday, with the World Trade Center rescue and recovery effort fully operational, we had 639, including three bones.

My worst fears had materialized. My head was swimming with things I had to do, and the phone never stopped ringing. I often had my desk phone in one ear, my cell phone in the other, while my secretary, Ashie Henry, was also delivering messages. Howard Baum reminded me that we needed freezers. I called Lorraine Kelly, our procurement assistant commissioner, and ordered two low-temperature Revco models. One of the first questions I had to consider was: how would they get into the city? New York was closed to the outside world.

Getting the freezers into the city and buying them were two separate issues. I always thought that the New York City procurement system should have required a doctorate in some appropriate discipline, a minor in psychology, and courses in anger management. It reminded me of a crotchety old man who delighted in confounding, confusing, and tormenting his best friends. City employees ordering supplies and equipment automatically became its de facto enemies.

I learned to hold my breath after placing purchase orders for almost anything because I knew they had embarked on an uncertain, circuitous path that could take months or years. Strangely, some orders made it through quickly. Others never made it at all. After

September 11, things changed. Although swamped with work, perpetually understaffed, and unappreciated, Lorraine Kelly's OCME procurement group processed the agency's orders immediately and got them through the system in record time. To the city's credit, it responded quickly, too. I had the freezers on Friday, September 14.

As early as Wednesday, September 12, I was feeling the pressure, mostly self-imposed, to start the DNA testing. It had already become a hot topic, and I knew it was only a matter of time until the mayor's staff would be demanding statistics: how many samples had we received? How many of the remains had we extracted for DNA? How many DNA profiles had we generated?

I considered asking Chuck Hirsch if we could hold off until we had an electronic tracking system. I knew his answer would be no. I believed, though it wasn't practical, that waiting to begin the DNA testing would have been wise. Instead, we were satisfying a personal need to be active, albeit at a huge risk. The DNA testing did not need to be rushed. We had time to install the proper systems to ensure that the effort would not be compromised. Waiting might have given us more time to plan and eliminate many of the problems we faced later on.

In those chaotic, early days when I was feeling the pressure to begin testing, I came to realize how important DNA would be for identifying most of those who died. The politicians, the media, and the World Trade Center families would eventually realize it, too, and focus on it. Such scrutiny made the work that much more difficult.

By Wednesday, the staff was working 24/7. My assistant directors divided the lab into two parts: disaster teams that focused on the World Trade Center effort and casework teams that handled the everyday crime-related work. Not unexpectedly, the reorganization caused problems. Almost everyone wanted to work on the World Trade Center effort, and those assigned to working criminal cases were angry. I hope they realize now how important their efforts were in stabilizing the laboratory and that their contribution was as important as that of those on the disaster teams.

By Wednesday the disaster teams were in full swing, working two twelve-hour shifts accessioning, processing, and extracting DNA from specimens almost as quickly as they arrived. Lydia DeCastro wrote an e-mail to the lab hinting at the nascent undercurrent of unrest. She said that she loved everyone for wanting to help, but suggested patience, and if they wanted to pitch in, they could sign up for nights and weekends.

Lydia's group was busy with the up-front work: accessioning World Trade Center specimens and extracting the DNA from tissues. They had to store the bones because we did not yet have a strategy to analyze them. Lisa Desire's group was handling the back-end work: working with the DNA extracts from tissues from Lydia's group to produce DNA profiles. By Friday she had DNA extracts from 514 of the 639 specimens.

At first, the processing of World Trade Center remains went something like this: after an anthropological review, which entailed sorting through what came into the morgue to separate nonhuman remains and artifacts from human remains and to separate commingled remains, by Amy Mundorff, a team of medical examiners removed laboratory specimens from the remains, placed them into bar-code-labeled, orange-capped 50-milliliter centrifuge tubes, then placed those into a red transfer box. A written manifest, a log of the samples present, accompanied the red box. Someone from the DNA team retrieved the red box from the morgue and carried it to the DNA laboratory, where Lydia's disaster team accessioned the specimens into the lab. At first this was a manual process; team members entered the DM number manually onto a processing sheet and then placed the specimen-containing tubes into a rack for processing.

Since the majority of the lab specimens we received were too large to analyze as a single piece, the disaster team, working under benchtop fume hoods (we purchased these because, after a week, the odor from decomposing tissue was too intense), snipped approximately 3-millimeter-square samples from the larger specimens, and placed them into smaller, labeled 1.5-milliliter conical tubes called microcentrifuge tubes. The original, larger sample went back into the 50-milliliter centrifuge tube, which was frozen at -80°F. The disaster group extracted the DNA from the smaller specimen.

Maintaining two twelve-hour shifts seven days a week rapidly sapped the lab's resources. People were burning out, and we needed help. Luckily, during those first few weeks we had so many volunteers that I even had to turn away several who were willing to leave their jobs for a month or more in order to help. In her Friday, September 14 e-mail, Mecki Prinz recognized that many of us were fielding phone calls from classmates, former colleagues, friends, and family. She opined that it would be better if volunteers had a science background and warned that the smell would get worse.

Bianca Nazzaurolo, a sixth-floor disaster team member, wrote that her fiancé was a medical student at Columbia University and was going to try to round up volunteer med students for morgue duty. After sending an e-mail, he got an overwhelming response and thought that he could get about thirty people, mostly second- and third-year med students. He also got some scrubs for us. She concluded that her fiancé was not only wonderful, tall, dark, and handsome, but added that he cooked, too. They are married now.

In addition to accessioning and DNA extraction responsibilities, Lydia had to schedule the lab staff and volunteers from the New Jersey State Police crime laboratory system, who worked with us for almost a year. Medical students from NYU and Columbia University helped in the morgue, accessioned specimens, and processed samples in the lab.

Even with all the volunteers, by the end of the second week, Lydia was desperate for help. She asked if the Disaster Mortuary Operational Response Team (DMORT), a group funded by FEMA (Federal Emergency Management Agency; both are currently a division of the Department of Homeland Security), could be brought in to support the lab. DMORT was originally a group of funeral directors organized regionally and trained to respond to emergencies. The membership now comprises DNA experts, pathologists, dentists, and funeral directors who can handle all aspects of a disaster at the request of the local medical examiner. They must be requested by the local community. At the time, I really was naïve about what DMORT could or could not do. I posed the problem to Dave Schomburg, who arranged for them to work in the lab for two twelve-hour shifts each day. Once they arrived in New York, they stayed until May 2002. They were terrific.

According to the media, based on projections made by the Giuliani administration, the expected length of the rescue-recovery operation would be up to a year. This meant that I would eventually have to face the issue of deteriorating DNA in the remains. If the thousands of tissues we would receive were badly decomposed, I wondered how effective DNA testing would be in identifying people. These fears became reality too quickly. Within a couple of weeks, the tissues were showing signs of extensive decomposition.

The steady decline in tissue quality coincided with the mayor's and the media's growing interest in DNA. They were beginning to realize that most of the identifications would come as a result of DNA testing. It worried me because I knew that the DNA inside such rapidly decomposing tissue and bone would eventually be worthless. Because of DNA's heralded success in criminal cases, rescuers, politicians, the media, and the families had a preconceived idea that DNA was infallible. Frankly, DNA had achieved an aura of mystical proportions. Months later, Amy Mundorff told me that firefighters would stand around the autopsy table watching her sort through badly charred bones inside bunker gear, a firefighter's protective uniform, where there was little or no chance that DNA was present. They were convinced DNA would do the impossible. "DNA will identify him," they'd say. That was scary because with samples so badly degraded, the technology never could live up to the hype.

The corollary was: if the DNA failed to make identifications, the perception would be that I had failed. The fact was that I had no control over either the quality of the remains coming into the lab or how successful the recovery effort would eventually be. Either way, DNA might end up with a bad rap. These concerns, plus the enormity of our task, dragged me down, and I had trouble driving these negative thoughts from my mind. I scolded myself and hoped my staff hadn't noticed. If my fears and pessimism became too transparent, it might adversely affect my staff and my ability to lead them effectively. So I forced myself to keep my mind pointed forward. It was not easy.

The quality of the remains reflected the micro-environments of the World Trade Center rubble, and each had an effect, stabilizing or not, on the DNA. These effects were somewhat predictable, but the number of those missing who had been exposed to each micro-environment was unknown. This dictated how many people we would eventually identify. Although the buildings burned for three months, the heat itself should not have adversely affected the DNA to the point where it was unanalyzable. However, the combination of heat and moisture was a problem. Because water had been sprayed onto the pile to cool it so that the rescue-recovery effort could continue, I expected that the bodies trapped inside that environment would rapidly decompose and yield poor-quality DNA. This is what happened.

A subset of remains had been exposed only to heat. Aided by the dust from the pulverized cement, these remains dehydrated and mummified. The DNA in these remains was decent. Another subset of remains had been exposed to intense heat and were burned and/or extensively charred; that DNA was poor for making identifications. Yet another subset had been buried under the heat at the bottom of the rubble. These remains appeared little different than any exhumed body, and though the tissue had decomposed, the bones still contained decent DNA.

Generally, bone offers a protective barrier from the elements and protects DNA. The experience of my colleague Dr. Ed Huffine, who was in charge of the DNA laboratory that was working at the time on remains taken from the mass graves in Bosnia after the ethnic cleansing there in the 1990s, reported that the DNA in bones was often in good shape. Although the DNA taken from some of the bones was extensively degraded, generally it was in better shape than that taken from the surrounding tissue.

I also learned an important lesson from Amy Mundorff, the OCME staff forensic anthropologist. Amy is an energetic, highly principled forensic anthropologist hell-bent on carving her niche in the profession. She has an MS degree in anthropology and joined my staff in 1998 after Chuck Hirsch asked for a full-time forensic anthropologist. Before the World Trade Center attacks, she was responsible for identifying bones that were found in New York City. In these instances, she helped the police or FBI excavate the remains of people who had been murdered and then buried, such as in mob hits. Then she would help identify who the person was and work with the medical examiner to ascertain the cause and manner of death. Now she became concerned with separating remains from each other, and from nonhuman remains and artifacts. She also inspected the identified remains before they were returned to families just to be sure no mistakes had been made.

Depending on the amount of heat the bones are exposed to, they become a yardstick by which one can estimate whether usable DNA is present: charred (black) or calcined (white) bones cannot be expected to have much usable DNA; calcined bones are essentially cremains, or ash, and thus have been so extensively heated that they no longer contain organic matter. This means no DNA. I told her not to waste her or my lab's time sending calcined bones. I still wanted the charred ones, just to be certain that we had not missed anything.

The quantity of poor-quality DNA coming into the lab was disturbing. Equally disconcerting was the number of remains coming, which seemed to be escalating at an alarming rate. Extracting DNA from such large numbers of tissue presented a huge coordination, control, and sample-handling problem. The decomposition added a wrinkle that compounded the DNA extraction process, requiring more exacting procedures to retrieve whatever usable DNA was still present.

And then there were the bones. By the end of September, except for a few select cases, we had not even started on them.

Removing DNA from inside dried cells is something forensic DNA analytical laboratories perform routinely in criminal cases. Typically this evidence comes from physical evidence, such as clothing, crime scenes, and weapons. It's a simple, straightforward procedure that even the most inexperienced scientist, even a high school student, can perform properly.

Fresh human tissue contains a large amount of high-quality DNA, and extracting it from within the tissue matrix—although a bit more time consuming than extracting DNA from a bloodstain—is rather straightforward. A number of reliable methods exist, which typically rely on an organic procedure wherein a combination of two rather unpleasant chemicals—phenol and chloroform—form the basis of the extraction.

Decomposing tissue, however, offers its own peculiar challenge. It contains an abundance of the digestive enzymes that are released during decomposition and then either destroy the DNA or render it fragile and thus susceptible to extensive fragmentation during extraction. One common step in the extraction process is to release the DNA by digesting the protein in which it is trapped with an enzyme that specifically chews up proteins, a protease. In decomposing tissue, the digestion process yields a fibrous mush that is often difficult to handle.

On Wednesday, September 12, we began extracting tissues manually. I desperately needed a method that would eliminate the human element as much as possible to avoid the possibility of a sample mixup. I wanted an automated procedure, one that employed robotics.

Do not confuse the term "robotics" with *Star Wars'* R2-D2 robot, although my lab did name one of our robots R2-D2. The robots we used for DNA extraction are simply automated liquid-handling systems that perform simple, repetitive laboratory chores such as pipetting—transferring—a sample from one tube or tray to another tube or tray. They also move tubes or trays from one place to another. Importantly, these systems easily process samples in a microtiter plate format. A microtiter plate is a plastic tray in which individual wells have been molded. Although a microtiter plate can hold anywhere from 48 to 1,536 samples, the most popular configuration is an 8 x 12-inch format that holds 96 individual samples.

On September 11, there was no robotic system in the DNA laboratory, although I had been trying to purchase one for several years. (The city's elusive procurement system had even approved one for funding, but I never saw it. Who knows what happened to it.)

On Wednesday, I was still shell-shocked from the World Trade Center events, groggy from working all night in the morgue, and not really paying attention when I answered the phone for what seemed like the millionth time. On the other end of the line Arne Masibay, a Promega Corporation sales and technical representative, wanted to offer his company's services. I don't know why his call made it through the innumerable ones coming in or why I even answered it—probably divine guidance.

Promega is a molecular biology company located in Madison, Wisconsin, that specializes in specialty reagents for, among other applications, forensic DNA analysis. Arne was the company's forensic representative, a knowledgeable and personable guy. Promega offers several forensic reagent packages used by the forensic laboratories in the United States. We adapted two for the World Trade Center DNA testing.

After the pro forma "How are you doing?" Arne asked to speak to either Howard Baum or Mecki Prinz. I had met Arne only once, at a dinner in Washington, DC, at the Second Annual NIJ Grantees Conference months earlier, so I doubted he remembered that I was the director of the lab. I probably sounded a bit brusque when I said, "I'm the one you have to talk to."

I was only half listening until he said something that captured my attention: "The IQ system runs on a Biomek 2000 platform." The Biomek 2000 is one of Beckman Instrument's robotic platforms. The

IQ system is Promega's DNA-extraction system. At the time, the IQ system was new and not yet accepted by most forensic scientists. Now I was all ears. According to Arne, Promega had successfully extracted DNA from tissue using the new robotic extraction system. It sounded like the IQ system fit perfectly with our World Trade Center needs.

When I hung up, my gut instinct was to purchase the IQ system immediately. I'm not certain whether it was Arne's reassurance that the IQ system would work, Promega's reputation, or just wishful thinking, but I needed a robotic system. Good or bad, I felt we had to make it work. Continuing to do the extractions manually was asking for trouble. I wondered if it would work with decomposing tissue. Fresh tissue and decomposing tissue were distinct entities, each having unique characteristics. Since we had no experience with the IQ system, I was also concerned with how long it would take to get the system up and running.

Needing someone to temper my enthusiasm, I queried Howard Baum on his thoughts on the IQ system. Howard was the consummate skeptic who rightfully questioned Arne's claim. He harbored doubts that the IQ system would ever work.

Validating the system—making sure it would work—would take time. With specimens streaming into the laboratory, we had precious little. My optimistic side realized that the IQ system had to prove itself using decomposing tissue. If I succumbed to my impulse and began using the system straight out of the box, it might prove disastrous.

We formed yet a third disaster team, the IQ validation team, which Mecki headed. She recruited Dr. Theresa Caragine and Chris Kamnik to set up the validation experiments, which she hoped would be completed in a week. A week sounded optimistic, even for someone like me who was continually pressing forward.

The IQ system and the robots arrived 9/19.

Promega's development team installed the IQ system in the laboratory and then worked with my staff for the first week. Thereafter, they assisted via phone from their headquarters in Madison. As luck would have it, Murphy smiled wickedly at us.

By October 2, Mecki's frustration peaked. The validation process had escalated into a huge project and time sink, and there were moments when I wondered whether we'd ever get it working properly. Sometimes I even cursed my decision to buy it.

The IQ robotic system had become the proverbial albatross. Daily, it seemed, I had to report bad news to Chuck Hirsch. Like me, he was frustrated by the seemingly incessant delays. At times, the problems seemed intractable. First, the IQ digestion method didn't work with decomposing tissue. Then the robot caused problems. Experiment after experiment failed. We were spending too much time on the system, but I pushed Mecki to get it done.

Meanwhile, the disaster team continued extracting the tissues manually. It wasn't that the IQ system didn't generate good-quality DNA—it did. But the engineering on the robotic platform seemed all wrong. Initially, we tried extracting the maximum number of samples possible, which meant 88 samples adjacent to each other on the microtiter plate.

Each variation resulted in failure, as the robot disturbingly cross-contaminated them. It was an intolerable situation. In desperation, Mecki changed her approach. Instead of extracting 88 adjacent samples simultaneously, she reduced the number to 44, leaving a blank space between each sample. We called this a checkerboard pattern. It worked like magic. The checkerboard approach eliminated the cross-contamination. Although our output was cut in half, I didn't care. We had a robotic extraction system online for extracting DNA. The DNA was clean and contaminant free, and having the extraction system functional meant that the disaster team would have time for other chores.

It took almost exactly a month to bring the IQ process online; but the IQ validation did not end. Theresa Caragine spent the next eight months optimizing it for what turned out to be Phase II of the World Trade Center project, when we had to go back and reextract thousands of samples.

• • •

Right from the beginning, we had also needed a way to obtain STR profiles from extracted remains quickly. Luckily, Applied Biosystems (ABI) had recently released a capillary electrophoresis (a technique for separating DNA fragments) system, the 3100, which analyzed sixteen samples every forty-five minutes.

I spoke to the Applied Biosystems sales representative and ordered two instruments. My administrative assistant spoke on Wednesday to the director of genetic technologies at Applied Biosystems, who told her that the 3100s would be in the air by 9/13.

Cortney Boccardi, who was a criminalist in my lab and is now a scientist at the New Jersey Bureau of Forensic Science, e-mailed me on 9/12 that the 3100s would be in White Plains, New York, at 1:00 P.M. the next day. At that time, the FAA (Federal Aviation Administration) had stopped all commercial air travel. The only air traffic was military. Chuck Hirsch wrote to the FAA requesting permission to have the instruments flown into New York. His request was rejected. Although the company is in Foster City, California, it had instruments in North Carolina. These were driven to White Plains, where I arranged for a police escort to get them into New York City. They arrived at the laboratory on Friday, 9/14.

Although it was a chaotic time, we managed to keep our laboratory traditions intact. One was the naming of new instruments. As Mecki wrote on Friday, September 14, we had to name the new arrivals. Many interesting possibilities were suggested, but Stars and Stripes stuck.

Applied Biosystems placed a team of specialists in the lab to set up the machines and help us validate them for the World Trade Center disaster samples. Validating a scientific procedure means performing a series of experiments designed to show that a specific method gives reliable test results in the circumstance in which it will be used. It was another validation project, and I was leery of it. I didn't doubt that the instruments worked, but I was again concerned about the time it would take to get them up and running.

• • •

Next I had to consider how, or if, we could continue working the routine homicide and sexual assaults. Although we had suspended the work temporarily on September 11, we had to get back to that work soon. I discussed our options with Chuck Hirsch. One thought was to outsource our regular caseload to vendors. We had been working with private laboratories to analyze seventeen thousand backlogged rape cases that had accumulated in the NYPD's property clerk's office since 1990. We reasoned it might be possible to piggyback current cases onto that contract.

After some discussion, we agreed that sending our routine criminal cases to private laboratories was not in the long-term best interests of the city. However, until we had a better alternative, it remained a possibility. Another thought was for the laboratory to accept a more minor role, as yet undefined, in the World Trade Center work. Certainly, rapists and murderers would not remain on holiday for long, though two weeks passed before the first rape was reported in Manhattan after the attacks.

A couple of weeks after September 11, and after Chuck Hirsch and I met to discuss our casework situation, Dr. Jennifer Smith called. At the time, Jenny was the head of the FBI's DNA laboratory in Washington, DC. She wanted to know how the FBI could help us with the World Trade Center work.

During our conversation after September 11, I said that having the FBI accept a certain percentage of our rape cases would help dramatically. I never considered sending them all, perhaps a third or only about six hundred cases. Jenny seemed less than enthusiastic, but like a good friend, she agreed to run it by her bosses. I never heard anything back from the FBI.

The outcome of the conversation was that we would continue analyzing criminal cases that required DNA analysis. In October, Marie Samples wrote an e-mail explaining that we would accept evidence from rapes and homicides. The schedule would run from Monday to Friday instead of seven days a week. She anticipated that the laboratory rotations responsible for signing in evidence and examining it would ramp back up to their normal volume before long.

• • •

The World Trade Center work created a skyrocketing need for supplies, which thrust procurement into a prominent role. We needed more of everything, and we had to order things we had rarely used before, such as dry ice. The lab was beginning to operate at a feverish pitch, which was escalating. Thankfully, I had someone in the lab who had been keeping track of our procurement activity.

When Joselyn Cherwnjawski, a supervising criminalist, speaks, her voice is soft, and she lifts her chin and appears to speak to heaven. Honestly, I'm not sure what the New York City cop wife stereotype should be, but whatever it is, to me, it isn't Joselyn.

In addition to her DNA laboratory casework responsibilities, she also handled our laboratory's purchasing requirements. After September 11, she transformed herself into an in-lab World Trade Center miracle worker. She kept us afloat and worked closely with Lorraine Kelly and Joanne Valentine in procurement to keep supplies flowing. Because of her, the work continued. She also tracked spending for the Federal Emergency Management Administration (FEMA), which meant that she had to keep tabs on spending that would eventually be reimbursed.

It was a difficult, frantic time for all of us. But everyone pulled together. Petty bickering and complaining ceased, and the kindness and generosity of the human spirit shone brightly. For example, Bianca wrote to the lab on Friday, 9/14, that she had an extra pair of socks and a nonvegetarian lunch available.

And through it all, there was humor. A newspaper article about Vice President Cheney's pacemaker problems and subsequent hospitalization sparked DNA scientist Carole Meyers's imagination. She joked in an October e-mail, "As you know, Dick Cheney has been removed to a remote location for safety purposes. Just between you and me, he's at my apartment and he is doing just fine. No heart problems as of this morning, and, believe me, after a night like last night, he can withstand anything. No pacemaker problems, either."

A couple of days later, her humorous e-mail picked up where it left off, "This is a Cheney update. Dick is doing very well and he is very relaxed and happy. I accidentally turned on the microwave while he was in the kitchen and he went into v-fib. I de-fibbed him and gave him mouth to mouth for a really very long time and he's better than new now. Nothing else to report at the moment, but we are hoping for some little Cheneys in the near future."

4 A STRATEGY EMERGES

September 14, 2001

Number identified: 35

DNA-Only identifications: 0

When Mark Dale called from the New York State Police Forensic Investigation Center on Wednesday, September 12, I had been completely immersed in keeping my emotions in check and my head on straight. I really hadn't thought about the New York State Police and whether they could or would help. My mind had not yet taken me that far. My prevalent thoughts ranged from tracking samples, extracting them, and preparing the lab to analyze human remains to staffing morgue shifts and dealing with the media and the mayor's staff.

From within that chaotic milieu, Mark Dale's voice hit me like a loud foghorn in a dense fog, a welcome sound, a drowning sailor's delight. He and Dr. Barry Duceman, the DNA laboratory director for the New York State Police, had been assessing the New York State Police DNA laboratory's capacity. Although it did not register at that exact moment, the way he had phrased the question later stuck fast to my thoughts. "Would you mind if I contact the other public labs to find out what extra capacity there might be out there?"

In the early 1990s Barry Duceman and I were struggling to build credible forensic DNA laboratories. Though friendly rivals, ours was a spirited competition to see who could build the biggest and most productive lab. Barry even said once that when he met with Howard Baum, it felt like it was a constant game of one-upmanship.

Barry's a bright and knowledgeable guy who obtained his PhD from Pennsylvania State University and came to the state police from the New York State Department of Health. As directors of two of the largest public forensic DNA laboratories in the country, Barry and I often met to commiserate about our problems and to relish our successes. Although we usually found ourselves on the same page with respect to most emerging issues, we differed about mitochondrial DNA typing as it should be applied to the World Trade Center effort. Mitochondrial DNA, or mtDNA, is circular and located inside the mitochondria of a cell. It is maternally inherited and, while useful to track maternal lineage, it is not necessarily unique. Different from nuclear DNA, which is typically employed in forensic testing, it has been used to aid in identifying human remains.

During most of the World Trade Center work, Barry's direct supervisor was Inspector Mark Dale, then the director of the Forensic Investigation Center in Albany, which housed the New York State Police DNA laboratory, the Biological Sciences Unit. Mark is the director of the Northeast Regional Forensic Science Initiative after a stint as the director of the New York City Police Department laboratory. I've known Mark Dale for years. As members of the New York Crime Laboratory Advisory Committee, a committee of New York's crime laboratory directors and other law enforcement groups, we often philosophized about and discussed laboratory management issues with an eye toward improving forensic services in the state.

In his fifties, though appearing much younger and athletic, Mark usually wears a dark suit, a white shirt, and a power tie. His ruddy, round baby face, piercing blue eyes, and engaging smile mask a quick, independent mind and sharp wit. On Friday, 9/14, when he and his boss, Bill Callahan—the director of the Forensic Investigation Center in Albany—came to the OCME, I did a double take because Mark was out of uniform, wearing a New York State Police pullover and jeans.

Mark's experience as a crime laboratory administrator for both the New York State Police and the Washington State Patrol became quickly apparent; he likes to solve problems, and his mind always works toward that end in the form of interagency cooperation. It didn't come as a complete surprise when he proposed a joint OCME–New York State Police DNA effort for the World Trade Center disaster.

A couple of years earlier when Mark and I first discussed various aspects of mass-disaster management (after Ron Forney had presented his account of how the Royal Canadian Mounted Police had handled the 1998 Swissair crash), I suggested to him and Barry that we form an alliance or network of public labs to share the onerous responsibility of performing DNA tests. It might have meant the capacity for analyzing thousands of samples. Like Mark, I thought the state's DNA laboratories could split testing responsibilities in a disaster, such as a plane crash. I certainly believed, correctly it turned out, that a mega–mass fatality of any size could quickly overwhelm any single public forensic laboratory. Mark and Barry had agreed, but nothing happened.

Mark's question on Wednesday was completely in character, and I immediately chastised myself for not remembering my own thinking on the subject. Mark has always been a thoughtful strategist, and I was thankful that someone's mind was working clearly.

Mark believed that if we distributed the workload as much as possible between the OCME and the New York State Police, the burden on my lab would ease. I'm certain he felt, like we all did, a need to be involved.

Interestingly, I experienced a fleeting pang of paranoia when Mark mentioned assessing *their* capacity and his plan to distribute the work between the agencies. I couldn't help think that high-level discussions had already decided who should be directing the World Trade Center DNA effort. I felt threatened. Who would steal the responsibility from my lab?

These thoughts took me back to January 2000, when New York

State officially became a part of the national DNA database called the Combined DNA Index System, or CODIS. Apparently someone at the Division of Criminal Justice Services decided that my laboratory had a number of crime-scene DNA profiles that, by uploading them into CODIS, would be impressive politically. The state wanted DNA profiles in the newly created state DNA database (the state's part of the FBI's national DNA data-bank system, CODIS). There was one problem. The state didn't have DNA profiles to put into the data bank; the vast majority of forensic DNA profiles theoretically available resided in my laboratory. Certainly, no other state laboratory had a meaningful number of casework DNA profiles.

My lab had always been one of the more progressive in the country. We also had had a functioning, albeit non-CODIS, local DNA database since 1996. These DNA profiles, however, existed in a format that was not acceptable to the FBI. Regardless, the pressure to get these DNA profiles into CODIS was intense. What those at the state did not know was that in order to enter the data into CODIS, my laboratory had to rework more than nine hundred cases. This set the laboratory back, creating a monumental casework backlog and an unacceptably large turnaround time.

Unfortunately, this happened when the lab staff had been working diligently to lower our turnaround time and case backlog. Our turnaround time for routine homicide and sexual assault DNA cases had fallen from ninety-three to sixty-six days, and my staff was beginning to swagger. I was proud of what we had accomplished.

Things went from bad to worse. At the same time, we had our annual accreditation inspection and had scheduled a bloodstain pattern interpretation course for nearly one-third of the staff. What happened was predictable. The pressure increased immeasurably, which nearly destroyed me and my staff. Our turnaround time and case backlog skyrocketed. The new turnaround time peaked at 208 days in December 2000, which attracted the attention of the mayor's office.

The mayor's criminal justice coordinator demanded a series of high-level meetings about the DNA laboratory that included Chuck, Deputy Commissioner for Administration Tom Brondolo, Counsel to the Chief Medical Examiner Sarah Scott, me from OCME, the New York City Police Department, and representatives from all five borough district attorneys' offices. In the end, the city wanted a thirty-day turnaround time on all DNA rape cases and asked me to develop a plan to make it happen. I had to comply. Implementing it stressed and demoralized my entire staff. By the beginning of September 2001, although our turnaround time had fallen to fifty-five days, the entire staff was walking on eggshells. We were exhausted.

As I listened to Mark's proposal on Wednesday, September 12, I was silently questioning whether the same insidious forces were working yet again. But why would an inspector of the New York State Police ask my permission for anything? He had asked if I *minded* whether he and Barry assessed the capacity of other public forensic labs. How bizarre! Then it hit me. He was offering to contact other labs on *my* behalf, tacitly acknowledging that the DNA effort for the World Trade Center was my responsibility, no one else's.

It's a good thing I was sitting down. I remember shutting my eyes and taking a deep breath. A chill coursed through my body. For the first time, I had a conscious doubt. Could I pull this off?

Analyzing samples received from the World Trade Center site was only half of the overall identification process. The other half involved analyzing the DNA obtained from families. These samples were of two kinds, both important. Shiya Ribowsky refers to these as antemortem DNA as opposed to DNA obtained from postmortem specimens. There are two types of antemortem DNA samples collected: material from biological relatives of the missing victims (usually buccal [mouth] swabs) and DNA of the missing people obtained from their toothbrushes, hairbrushes, razors, and biopsy specimens, to name a few sources.

On Wednesday, 9/12, Marie Samples and Karen Dooling visited the Family Assistance Center at New York University Medical

School, a temporary collection spot set up in the immediate aftermath of the attacks, to drop off family samples that had mistakenly been delivered to the medical examiner's office by an anonymous person. They were also curious to learn about the Family Assistance Center operation and thought it would be important to understand the process. They met Red Cross staffers who were working with NYPD personnel. What they found was appalling.

Grieving family members were filling out a seven-page questionnaire by hand and supplying a photograph of a missing person. The form had information about the missing person, such as physical characteristics—including scars, tattoos, birthmarks, injuries, workplace address, relatives, and jewelry and clothing worn. Eventually, the paperwork and photographs would be transferred to the OCME records unit.

Marie and Karen were concerned that the premature collection of DNA "exemplars" (antemortem DNA) might be disruptive. They knew that maintaining consistency between the manually completed forms, which would eventually be transcribed into an electronic version, would be impossible. Marie realized that someone would eventually have to collect oral swabs and personal effects from the families, and that someone, probably someone in the lab, would match the paperwork to swabs and personal effects from family members to a remain. No one was ensuring that this information would end up in the proper place and in the proper format.

Marie has the uncanny ability to correctly size up any situation and instantly zero in on its fatal flaw. At the Family Assistance Center, she recognized that the New York City Police Department's procedures were the genesis of a nightmare.

Not everyone who died at the World Trade Center was a New Yorker. Many came from outside the city's five boroughs and many were foreign nationals. So what about the families who did not live in the New York metropolitan area? How did their personal effects and kinship samples get into New York City and then to the testing laboratories? We needed a way to establish Family Assistance Centers across the world.

The New York City Police Department needed written guidelines for collecting family samples. They recognized—sadly, too, I'd guess—that the only forensic genetic expertise in the city resided in my laboratory. So the pressure came from Chuck Hirsch, who put Howard Baum under the gun to write the guidelines and also to line up an antemortem DNA collection facility for out-of-town families. Early Thursday evening, Howard was still waiting for Lab Corp to approve using their 900 nationwide parentage collection centers. When approval finally came, he hastily prepared a one-page kinship form for the NYPD so that police officers could collect antemortem DNA from family members. Howard intended the kinship form to be a guide because, in reality, it required some understanding of genetics and parentage testing in order to use it properly. On Thursday afternoon, no one knew who would staff the Family Assistance Center or collect the antemortem DNA samples. Logically, someone knowledgeable about DNA testing, genetics, and which samples to collect for kinship analysis should have been present. This person could answer questions or explain the DNA process to the families, who would be giving samples on blind faith. I wanted the process to go smoothly and, most important, correctly. I assigned Pasquale "Pat" Buffolino to the Family Assistance Center.

Pat sent an e-mail that said, in part, that the collection of family samples would take place at the Lexington Avenue Armory between Twenty-sixth and Twenty-seventh Streets. He wrote further that he would be at work on Friday morning to instruct the nursing staff on how to collect oral swabs for DNA testing. The family center collection process rapidly became unnecessarily complicated. Pat's frustration was apparent when he said that the entire process had been changed three times by the NYPD since being informed of the project.

Good to his word, though, Pat was ready on Friday morning. He had prepared a box that contained everything he needed to collect samples from family members. This meant we would soon begin seeing DNA profiles from the family samples, which meant we would start making identifications.

"The best laid plans . . ." Well, Pat Buffolino never had the opportunity to collect either personal effects or kinship swabs. On Thursday morning, before Pat was to staff the armory, the NYPD wrested control of the entire Family Assistance Center operation from our hands. Actually, it was more like an edict.

At least that's how it felt. I certainly did not have the clout, but I wanted to scream, "This isn't how it's supposed to be done," or "This is inviting disaster." Right or wrong, the New York City Police Department took over. The cops thrust police officers into a situation for which they were ill prepared. That's how I felt then and it's how I still feel. In hindsight, it was both a good and bad decision.

The police officers who collected the samples had no training or the appropriate educational background in kinship analysis, DNA testing, or genetics. It's not surprising that many of the samples they collected were inappropriate. For them, it was mission impossible! To their credit, the officers followed their orders and did the best they could under trying circumstances, although clearly they were not suitable for that job.

Needless to say, I was furious. I hated the strong-arm tactics, which I considered typical of the NYPD guarding its perceived turf. Privately, I was thankful for not having the responsibility. The World Trade Center attacks were only two days old, and my staff and I were overwhelmed. Adding the family specimen collection responsibility, although logically the proper thing to do, would have exacerbated the stress and likely would have produced errors.

In reality, it should have been a joint project and planned in advance. The medical examiner/coroner in any locality has and should have complete responsibility for making identifications in mass-fatality events and should work proactively with the families, law enforcement, and an emergency management agency. On September 11, most medical examiners didn't get it. They still believe their responsibility began and ended in calling the FBI and DMORT and in performing autopsies.

When politicians, police, and medical examiners figure out what we learned—mass fatalities are all about families—they might get it right. Working with the families is critical to getting the job done properly, and the truth is that the medical examiner and the police need to establish a synergistic relationship from the outset and then cooperate. The police and fire departments are typically responsible for the rescue efforts and for controlling and collecting physical evidence; this might also be an FBI responsibility, depending on the nature of the disaster. Then the medical examiner takes over and might also be responsible for the recovery effort. The Family Assistance Center is where the samples are collected that will be used to make identifications. Since the medical examiner is responsible for making the identifications, he should assume the responsibility for the Family Assistance Center, while geneticists and/or forensic biologists—most likely the DNA lab staff, which might be a part of the police department—should be available to assist.

My DNA staff had been excluded, which meant we had little input (except for Howard's kinship sheet) in determining which samples were collected or how they were packaged and cataloged. The collection was done manually, which was a mistake, because no one in New York City's law enforcement community had the capability to track the family personal effects or kinship swabs electronically. In the end, it created a mess for my lab when we needed accurate metadata (the data from all sources except for DNA).

Okay, it's confession time.

I didn't have sufficient staff to do the job properly, which would have required me to allocate personnel twelve hours a day for months. The police did it, and considering the chaos of the time, did a splendid job. This isn't fingerpointing. It's simply a lesson learned. Many of the police officers, themselves grieving lost comrades, had to interview and collect evidence from grieving families. It was an enormously draining task.

I had become so completely immersed in the DNA effort, I didn't have much time to think about how many the OCME had identified.

However, by the close of the day on Friday, September 14, the OCME had identified thirty-five people. None by DNA.

Friday, September 14, proved to be a pivotal day, one that would define the World Trade Center DNA effort for months. The meeting with Mark Dale, Barry Duceman, and Bill Callahan was in Chuck's office. From Mark's call on Wednesday, I already knew the gist of his message, but I listened intently as he outlined his plan to divide the World Trade Center responsibilities.

Mark suggested having the DNA laboratory at the New York State Forensic Investigation Center assume responsibility for the family kinship samples and the personal effects, which the families of missing loved ones were bringing to NYPD collection points in the city. I was surprised when he admitted that the New York State Police DNA lab did not have the capacity to do additional DNA testing beyond their regular casework. He also surprised me by proposing shutting down the state DNA database and converting that space into a personal-effects examination laboratory so that the New York State Police could accept family samples from the NYPD, catalog them, and accession (extract DNA from) the personal effects.

This was huge! My mind immediately backtracked to a year and a half earlier when the state caused me and my laboratory so much grief over getting STR profiles into the state's forensic DNA database.

Mark's plan called for the New York State Police DNA lab to extract DNA from the personal effects and send the DNA extracts to a private laboratory; he was suggesting Myriad Genetics in Salt Lake City, Utah. He also recommended sending the oral swabs collected from family members directly to Myriad, which would extract the DNA and then run the routine forensic STR tests on both the DNA extracts from the personal effects and on the family swabs. Myriad would send the STR data to the New York State Police in Albany.

The agreement we made on September 14 with the state police to share Myriad Genetics Laboratory for DNA testing services made sense. The state police had an existing contract with Myriad to do

STR testing on convicted felons' blood and saliva for input into CODIS. Also, the STR test produces data that the FBI accepts for the national DNA network, the system that is so efficient at identifying serial murderers and rapists. It is also the same test employed in my laboratory and at the New York State Police for our routine criminal casework. This should have made our effort easier, since we were familiar with the data format, its peculiarities, failings, and shortcomings.

We struck the deal. The New York State Police would handle the family samples, which meant I could eliminate that problem from my list. My laboratory could concentrate on extracting the DNA from the victims. We would send the extracts to Myriad. This also meant that my laboratory could go back to concentrating on casework and my instruments would not be tied up by the World Trade Center testing.

After Myriad returned the data to Albany, the New York State Police would import the STR data, error check it, and then somehow get it to us. At that time, it was only guesswork as to how that would happen. Karen Dooling had ongoing discussions with the FBI concerning setting up a stand-alone CODIS network between Albany and New York City.

My personal role also changed. In addition to having the responsibility for the city's casework DNA laboratory, I had also become the manager of the World Trade Center DNA work. Under Mark's plan, I thought that I would no longer have to worry about having my laboratory perform the World Trade Center DNA testing. Instead, I would direct the DNA testing from afar. I could keep a finger on the pulse of the routine casework and also manage the World Trade Center work.

By agreeing to the split, I felt I had given away some of my responsibility. Strangely, an irrational part of me still wanted to do it all. So did my lab staff. When I told them about our agreement with the state police, many took offense. Several expressed outright anger. Like me, they suspected someone had pulled the plug on us.

Many even thought it meant that the mayor had lost faith in us, which was not true.

Myriad's reputation as a high-volume, fast-turnaround testing laboratory was unsurpassed in the industry. Additionally, it was a well-recognized genetics company that holds patents on the breast cancer genes. It operates a state-of-the-art robotic format for its STR DNA testing. Importantly, this was the same type of DNA testing my laboratory was running on World Trade Center samples and on routine casework, and that made interpreting data easier for my staff. It also meant that the DNA testing could be done faster and, we hoped, identifying the missing could be done much quicker than if my lab assumed the entire testing burden.

Under Mark's plan, my laboratory retained the responsibility for the remains collected at the World Trade Center site. We were already extracting DNA from the World Trade Center tissues and had begun STR testing. Our deal with the state police allowed us to piggyback onto its contract and send these DNA extracts from the remains to Myriad. Almost overnight, Myriad had assumed what seemed at the time the responsibility for the bulk of what I call Phase I of the STR DNA testing, at least for the analysis of the DM tissues and family samples.

I hadn't thought about it on Friday, September 14, but the New York State Police deal complicated my management role. Now I had three organizations to orchestrate. While that was somewhat disconcerting, partnering with the state police and Myriad made sense. This would mark the beginning of a continually expanding OCME DNA effort.

Two weeks before September 11, the State Police Forensic Investigation Center went "live" with their new laboratory information system, or LIMS, called the BEAST in their DNA laboratory. The BEAST is an evidence-tracking system available from Porter-Lee Corporation. Tim Smith, president of Porter Lee, agreed to have the

New York State Police install the BEAST in my laboratory so that we could track and control the World Trade Center remains coming into the laboratory. Was this another divine sign?

From day one, each of the remains coming into the DNA laboratory had a bar-code label stuck onto its 50-milliliter orange-capped plastic centrifuge tube. However, these were useless tags because we did not have bar-code readers with which to read them. A New York State Police team came to the laboratory in the third week of September and installed the BEAST and several bar-coding stations. They trained my staff, and we began using the system to track samples coming into the lab. Finally, some of the important pieces of the World Trade Center puzzle were falling into place.

We had three thousand remains by the end of the third week in September, all of which had been accessioned manually. These had to be put into the electronic system. My staff was swamped. So, while the sixth-floor disaster team accessioned the incoming remains, state police personnel went back to those original remains and put them into the system.

5 ALL THOSE BONES

Forensic bone analysis is the least enjoyable yet most challenging analytical task facing DNA scientists. Aside from the bones' almost sweet, unpleasant odor, simply handling another person's bones seems almost like an invasion of privacy. I'm not sure why, but I usually shiver or feel uncomfortable when I pick up a human bone to examine it. Maybe it's simply that after we die, our bones are the last remaining physical vestige of who we once were. Even the extreme prolonged heat of the World Trade Center fires did not totally destroy them, although some had become white cremains, a constant reminder of that hellish day.

Bones are a critical component of the identification process. They, along with teeth and possibly hair, are the most reliable source of non-commingled DNA available. For the World Trade Center work, especially, tissue proved to be the most unreliable DNA source because of commingling.

DNA is found inside of cells called chondrocytes, which are trapped within the bony matrix. This matrix protects the DNA somewhat from detrimental environmental insults and makes bone an excellent source of DNA from decomposing bodies. It also complicates the DNA extraction process. Most forensic DNA laboratories have a DNA bone procedure. And while each has its own nuances, most follow a series of similar steps.

First, the scientist must remove all surface contamination, usually by scraping or sanding. Because bone is a porous matrix, the first few millimeters of the bone can absorb tissue, which might come from decomposing tissue, so it must be removed. This is especially a problem where commingling is expected in those instances when two people die together.

Many of the bones coming into the DNA laboratory were recovered by the medical examiner from larger remains at the time of the autopsy. These had adhering tissue that had to be removed. Many bones unattached to a specific body part were found at the World Trade Center site or the Staten Island Fresh Kills landfill, which was where WTC site rubble was taken and sifted through again on a conveyor belt to locate human remains. Of the bones brought to the laboratory, many had dried or had become charred and had adhering tissue contaminated with dirt and dust. The contamination had to be removed.

Second, using a bone saw, a sample of the bone's central core was obtained. In the case of long bones, the core is the bone marrow. Next, we pulverize the core into a powder using a mill filled with liquid nitrogen to keep the bone cold, as milling generates heat, which can affect the DNA. Once we have the bony powder, we subject it to an extended DNA extraction process that can take several days. The bone DNA extraction process is tedious and time consuming, and requires a special space in a ventilated hood to reduce the odor and dust.

As we moved into week three and beyond, the bones came into the laboratory in bunches. By the end of the first week, we had only 3 bones. On September 30, we had 631, and by October 8, we had 1,241, nearly double in eight days. The flow of bones into the laboratory was growing at an alarming rate.

How in the world would I get all of them analyzed?

Forensic bone analysis cannot be done by just any DNA laboratory. It requires a laboratory that has experience analyzing bones and, critically, experience with bones from decomposing bodies. The Armed Forces DNA Identification Lab was the logical choice. The scientists there have experience in mass-fatality investigations and, additionally, had been analyzing human bones for years in an effort to identify our nation's war missing. The Armed Forces DNA Identification Lab was already busy working on identifying those who died in the September 11 Pentagon and Pennsylvania crashes.

I seriously considered outsourcing the bone work to multiple public forensic laboratories or even a combination of private and public forensic laboratories. However, the more I thought about it, the less I liked the idea. How much of a commitment could a public laboratory promise given its responsibility to its jurisdiction? There was also an expense. Could a public forensic laboratory afford to donate the equipment, personnel, and costs required? Probably not.

Also, if I chose several public and/or private labs, tracking the samples would become a nightmare, a task that would fall into Lydia's lap.

Tracking the DMs was already complex, considering I had three laboratories—the New York State Police, my laboratory, and Myriad—in the pipeline. My lab was pretty much swamped with World Trade Center tissue DMs from which we were extracting DNA. By October 8, we had 3,038 muscle specimens in-house. The New York State Police was deluged by family samples with more to come, which left them out. Myriad did not process bones.

I needed a forensic lab that could analyze bone. I considered using my laboratory for some of the work, but I needed to know how much of the burden my laboratory would have to assume. I had to make a decision fast.

Pat Buffolino had recently completed his work on a World Trade Center bone extraction procedure, so I asked, "Pat, how many bones can we analyze in a week?"

He thought for a moment. Then he began listing the additional workstations we would need, the number of people we would have to assign to each workstation, and how many bones each workstation could process in a day. As I listened, I envisioned a horror in the making. My lab clearly did not have the space to set up eight new individual workstations. As much as I wanted us to handle the bones, my path seemed obvious. I asked again, "How many?"

He looked at me. "Maybe forty or fifty—a hundred."

That clinched it. At the rate bones were coming into the lab—the final number would approach 14,000—we would be analyzing bones for the next ten years. I doubted Mayor Giuliani, Chuck Hirsch, or the families would have considered it a viable plan. I decided that my laboratory would have nothing to do with the routine bone analysis.

Howard Baum and I started calling private forensic laboratories. I chose private forensic laboratories over public forensic laboratories because I could put them under contract. I had received a letter from Dr. Francis Collins offering National Institutes of Health help with the work. Again, as good as the NIH is, it is not a forensic organization, and I had doubts it would want to analyze these bones.

I needed a laboratory that understood the nuances of decomposing DNA and had experience with extracting DNA from charred bones. There was a caveat, too. The laboratory had to have the resources to begin analyzing immediately. It also had to have an STR-analysis procedure online that was CODIS compatible. I was looking for the proverbial needle in a haystack.

Near the end of September, Dr. Mitchell Holland, laboratory director of the Bode Technology Group in Springfield, Virginia, and now a professor at the Pennsylvania State University, visited New York. Bode was one of three private laboratories under contract to the city to process the NYPD's backlog of 17,000 rape kits. The purpose of Mitch's visit was to present data to us on the analysis of the sexual assault kits; he also offered to help with the World Trade Center work. At first, I did not believe the Bode group could help. Then I remembered that Mitch had worked for the Armed Forces DNA Identification Lab, which worked on the Alaska Airlines Flight 261 crash. An idea surfaced. Could Bode analyze the bones?

When I asked, I could almost hear the wheels grinding inside his head. He said, "Yes, but I'd like to discuss it with my staff."

The next day, Mitch called and said that they could process the bones. We still had to work out the details, but I was ecstatic with the general discussion.

A letter from Tom Bode Sr., general manager of the Bode Technology Group, to me on October 5 said they could handle approximately 250 bones per day, which translates into 1,250 a week or 5,000 a month.

I did not know Tom Bode very well, though I'd met with him on several occasions. I've always found him to be the consummate gentleman. Now retired, he's an almost-six-footer, thin-haired and sharp. Nothing gets by him, although his laid-back demeanor can be disarming. Most important, Tom is honest and he had put together a dream team of superb scientists whose forte was thinking out of the box.

I had learned this as part of a joint OCME Forensic Biology/New York City Police Department team that was looking for laboratories to analyze rape kits that the NYPD had in its evidence storage freezers going back almost a decade. What had impressed me was the way Bode attacked the problem. The original request specified a particular way in which samples were to be analyzed. Since these were rape kits, one step in the process was to identify semen. This was the conventional paradigm for analyzing rape kits, and thus it seemed like a no-brainer.

Bode took a different and unexpected tack. They reasoned they could achieve the same end faster and perhaps cheaper by looking for male DNA. Obviously, in a sexual assault case where the victim is female, male DNA is not necessarily supposed to be there. And that's the purpose of the testing: identify the male who left the semen. While it begs the question of the original allegation, I remembered this when I received Tom's letter saying they could process 250 bones a day. While the Bode approach to rape kit analysis might not have been better, it certainly was different.

I was not sure how Bode planned to approach the bone analysis, but my gut instinct assured me they would find a way. I also wondered whether I might need Bode's creativity again before we completed the World Trade Center DNA work, a thought that proved prophetic when we entered Phases II and III of the DNA testing.

On October 8, Bode's evidence clerk, Mark Radcliff, drove a van from Virginia to New York City armed with a letter from me granting him access to the city. No commercial vehicles were allowed into the city without an official reason. In fact, any vehicle entering Manhattan was subject to a search. He picked up approximately two thousand bones.

What Tom Bode did not explicitly say in his October 5 letter was that while the Bode group believed they could analyze 250 bones in a day, they had never done it. No one had. But they had an idea. Luckily for the World Trade Center families and for me, they delivered on their promise.

6 PHASE I: DNA TESTING

During that first week after the planes struck, I could only guess at how large the DNA-identification effort would become. But in order to allocate resources, I needed an estimate, even a ballpark one. The number two person in the OCME, Mark Flomenbaum, and I met with Chuck Hirsch on 9/12 to discuss the matter. Estimating the number of remains we would receive was not easy. Intellectually, we agreed that anyone inside those buildings likely had been pulverized into small fragments. The falling buildings had acted like two huge mortar and pestles, grinding the tissue and bone into smaller and smaller pieces, some of it to dust. The stark truth was that even normal office objects, such as computers and desks and chairs, were rarely found intact. Sadly people, too, had become tiny fragments that blended into the omnipresent dust that had become the hallmark of the World Trade Center rubble.

Mark pointed out that the human body has over two hundred bones, which meant that if we recovered every bone from everyone missing we could receive as many as a million samples, since early estimates were ranging as high as five thousand victims. While I doubted that would be the case, the number was overwhelming.

I had a sobering thought. What if we recovered only 10 percent of the remains? Given the projections of the number supposedly missing, that could translate into 100,000 remains: a lot. Based on what I knew about recovery rates from other mass disasters, 10 percent seemed reasonable. Recovering fewer would be hard to reconcile emotionally, as that meant many would be lost forever. I refused to allow myself to dwell on it.

We discussed how the grinding nature of the falling buildings would produce fragments much smaller than those usually recovered from mass disasters, such as air crashes. To err on the side of caution and to give ourselves a reasonable chance to identify as many as possible without analyzing every speck of dust, we decided to collect and DNA test everything that was at least the size of a thumb.

In an interview I did with Dr. Larry Altman of the *New York Times* on September 12, I speculated that we would receive approximately 20,000 samples. Then in another interview with another reporter, I guessed the number might be as high as 500,000. Who knew? My first estimate proved prophetic. The second was perhaps the result of a momentary panic attack, although the number had been mentioned when were trying to get a handle on a rough estimate.

Probably the only slam-dunk decision I made had to do with the specific test we would use. Everyone assumed we would use the same test we used for routine forensic casework: the STR test. It was the only completely reliable and U.S.-court-accepted forensic DNA test available. It was also used for the FBI's national DNA database, CODIS, and worldwide for criminal investigations. It had been successfully used in mass-fatality investigations, first by Dr. Jack Ballantyne, then a DNA section supervisor at the Suffolk County Crime Laboratory, for TWA Flight 800, which crashed off the coast of Long Island in 1998. We knew a lot about the STR test, its reliability, and suitability for mass-fatality investigations. As time went on, we learned even more.

The STR test is easy to perform, is adaptable to bulk processing of samples—also known as high-throughput testing—has semiautomated instrumentation, and works on degraded samples exposed to environmental insults, such as heat and humidity. For mass disasters, in addition to Flight 800, the Royal Canadian Mounted Police had used it successfully to identify the missing from the Swissair crash off the coast of Nova Scotia, and it was also used in the Alaska Airlines crash and the Waco, Texas, massacre. It is being used in London and Thailand, too.

In order to understand how identifications were made using DNA testing, it is important to illustrate what STR testing data looks like and how we used it to make IDs. The test offered many surprising twists and unexpected problems that we had to solve.

The STRs used for CODIS and for the World Trade Center investigations are found on the DNA located inside the nucleus of a cell, called genomic, or nuclear, DNA. Forensic scientists purposely chose to analyze STRs on different chromosomes in order to minimize the possibility that they were linked. Scientifically, this linking of genetic traits is called linkage disequilibrium, which creates problems when trying to ascertain the statistical strength of a kinship match. If the traits are not linked, they are considered statistically independent entities. If linked, they must be considered in groups, which complicates the calculation. For this reason, each STR employed in forensic testing is inherited independently. Using unlinked STRs makes these markers useful for performing kinship analysis.

The DNA inside the nucleus of our cells is inherited from our parents, with each contributing equal portions, so that half of our DNA comes from our mothers and half is from our fathers. While a complete STR profile tests 13 to 16 different regions of the DNA, we actually sample only a tiny fraction of the total DNA inside our cells.

A forensic STR test, such as the one employed in the World Trade Center work, is really a blend of up to 16 separate tests performed simultaneously. These DNA regions were chosen because they differ substantially from person to person such that, if a sufficient number of them type successfully, the result is a profile that is unique to an individual. For practical purposes, an STR profile containing as many as 13 regions, or loci, is unique. The only exception is identical twins, who have identical DNA profiles.

There are two basic mechanisms for identifying missing people using DNA. The easiest and quickest is called a direct match, where the STR profile from the remains is compared with the STR profile obtained from DNA on a missing person's personal effect, such as a toothbrush. If the two STR profiles are identical and if the probability that the two are from the same source meets predetermined statistical barriers—1 in 10 billion for the World Trade Center work—we safely concluded they came from the same person.

Table 1 illustrates the result of a hypothetical single STR test performed on a bone taken from the World Trade Center site and a toothbrush that belonged to someone who died there. The first column labeled "Locus" is the region (locus) of the DNA analyzed. In this instance, it is D3S1358. It tells us that the test was conducted on chromosome number 3, as represented by D3. The second column, "Bone," has two numbers: 14 and 16. These are numeric representations of genetic markers called alleles, which are actually STRs contributed to the person from each parent. For example, one parent donated version 14 of the D3S1358 STR to the son and the other parent donated version 16 of the D3S1358 STR. The child of these people will have both versions.

In order to make an identification, a sample that came from the missing person must have each of these present. The third column illustrates how the identification is made. In this instance, both the 14 and 16 versions (alleles) are present, which means there is a match at this locus. In order to make an ID, however, a sufficient number of regions must type successfully so that the appropriate statistical barrier is met.

TABLE 1. DIRECT MATCHING OF STR PROFILES

LOCUS	WORLD TRADE CENTER DM (BONE)	PERSONAL EFFECT (TOOTHBRUSH)
D3S1358	14, 16	14, 16

The numbers in the chart above are a scientist's interpretation of what is known as the underlying scientific data, or raw data. This is actually a graph called an electropherogram. An electropherogram is comprised of multiple peaks, shown in Figure 1, and is a printout of the original data as it comes from a genetic analyzer, a scientific instrument used in all forensic DNA laboratories. Each region of the DNA, a locus, will have one or two peaks. Each peak is an STR contributed by one parent. If only one peak is present, it means that both parents contributed the same STR to the child.

FIGURE 1. ELECTROPHEROGRAM

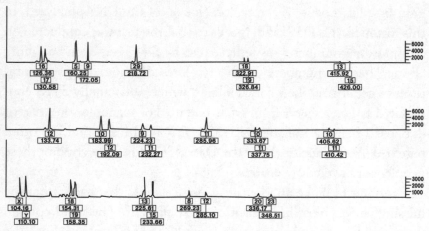

A scientist interprets the graph and determines what the digital representation of the peaks should be. In forensic casework, these numbers are coded digitally and then entered into the CODIS database. In the World Trade Center work, the numbers at each locus were compared directly.

A complete STR profile is much like the vehicle identification number assigned to each new automobile. It is a digital representation of the original DNA data on the electropherogram and might be looked at as a human identification number. As employed for law enforcement or the World Trade Center work, it tells us nothing about a person's predisposition to disease, physical traits, or ethnicity. In fact, Dr. Paul Ferrara, the director of the Virginia Bureau of Forensic Science, often shows a mocked-up Virginia driver's license that has his STR profile, which is simply the string of numbers printed under his picture. He challenges anyone to infer anything about him, his health, his race, or his physical characteristics. The list of numbers is uniquely his.

Another test employed for the World Trade Center effort was the identification of the amelogenin gene, which is found on both the X and Y chromosomes. A successful test result indicates the sex of an individual. If the test results showed only the X chromosome, the sample had to have come from a female. If testing showed contributions from the X and Y chromosomes, the sample was from a male.

A second method employs a technique called kinship analysis. This is simply a sophisticated paternity test in which we identify the genetic structure of the family and try to find remains that fit genetically. This works because of the inherited nature of DNA. A child's genetic makeup is inherited half from its mother and half from its father. An example of a hypothetical kinship match is shown in Table 2. Again, the D3S1358 locus is the example. In order to make a kinship identification, we had to be able to identify maternal and paternal contributions at each region of the DNA tested.

TABLE 2. KINSHIP MATCHING OF DNA PROFILES

LOCUS	MOTHER	WORLD TRADE CENTER SAMPLE (BONE)	FATHER
D3S1358	14, 15	14, 16	16, 16

In the table above, at the D3S1358 locus, all three STR profiles are different, which for kinship analysis isn't critical because we are not concerned whether the STR profiles match, but only that each parent contributes an STR (one allele) to his or her child at each locus. Here, the World Trade Center bone sample has a 14 and a 16 allele. If this bone truly came from their missing child, the parents must account for both of them, one from each. The mother has a 14 and the father has the 16. So at this single locus, kinship holds. However, in order to make the identification, kinship must hold at each locus. If true, we will have confirmed that the bone could be from their missing child. We had to prove that there was a 99.9 percent chance that these remains came from these parents (I'll talk about how we set that standard in chapter 10). Many times, we had probabilities lower than 99.9 percent and couldn't make the identifications. It was a troubling limitation of the work.

What if kinship didn't hold? In these instances, the World Trade Center sample would not fit into the family's genetic structure. The table below shows an example where the kinship does not hold. Notice that neither the mother nor the father has donated either the necessary 14 or 16 necessary to establish kinship.

TABLE 3. NONKINSHIP DNA PROFILE

LOCUS	MOTHER	WORLD TRADE CENTER SAMPLE (BONE)	FATHER
D3S1358	15, 15	14, 16	17, 17

Without making a single calculation, we quickly knew in this instance that the bone could not have come from their son.

Within a couple of weeks of September 11, the STR testing on World Trade Center remains began showing significant signs of DNA deterioration. In order to understand what we had to deal with, it is important to understand what degradation meant to us and how it affected our work. If the quality of the DNA had been good, we would have expected to obtain complete DNA profiles. We didn't.

DNA is a large molecule that resembles a twisted ladder. Each of its rungs is called a base pair, of which the DNA has approximately three billion. When DNA degrades, it progressively fragments until there is virtually no intact DNA remaining. The STR test we employed was specifically designed to analyze forensic samples where the DNA is often degraded. In fact, it is applicable to DNA that has fragmented to the point where only about four hundred of the three billion base pairs remain intact.

If the DNA had been of good quality, each of the thirteen to sixteen loci we tested should have given results. Additionally, the instrumental response to these samples at each locus should have given an electropherogram whose peaks were relatively even. That is, the peak heights at each locus should have been similar. In fact, most of the DNA we obtained from World Trade Center remains was degraded or was degrading, and the subsequent instrumental signal gave us peaks that were greatly unequal. Figure 2 is an electropherogram of degrading DNA.

The loci on the left have higher peaks, while those on the right are smaller. Since the fragment size of the loci increases as we move toward the right, the amount of DNA represented is progressively smaller. In this example, the DNA has not completely degraded. We know this because we are still getting a signal at each locus. Since each locus gave a positive test result, we could have used it to make an identification.

Each pair of peaks (sometimes a single peak) in the electropherogram represents one locus. In the electropherogram below, there are

FIGURE 2. DEGRADING DNA

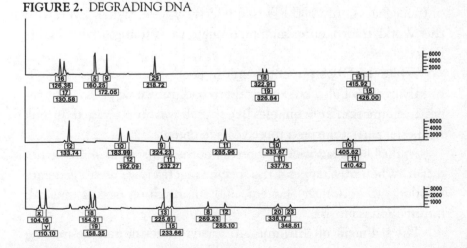

sixteen loci (the sixteen sets of numbers under the peaks). Notice the height of the first five peaks on the top row—these represent three loci. Notice how high and fairly constant the peaks are. Now examine the next four peaks, which represent two additional loci. The peaks are noticeably lower than the first five. The pattern of progressively smaller peak heights from left to right is the hallmark of degrading DNA.

The peak height is called the signal intensity, which is measured by an arbitrary scale expressed in reflectance units, or RFUs. This is a measure of the amount of DNA being analyzed. Small RFUs indicate small amounts of DNA. The instrument used to analyze STRs is normally set to "recognize" STRs at the minimum number of RFUs. If the DNA being analyzed has a small amount of DNA and the RFU is below the instrument's cutoff, the instrument will not "call," or record, it. In these instances, the data, although not lost, will not be reported. This became an issue as we moved deeper into the project.

The RFUs shown on the right side of the graph represent the amount of DNA "observed" by the instrument. In this instance, the intensity is as much as 6,000 RFUs, which is a strong signal.

The electropherogram opposite shows a different situation. Here, most of the STRs at most of the loci are gone. This type of electropherogram illustrates what we encountered often, and it represented badly degraded DNA. Only two loci have STRs, and the intensity of the signal is only 150 RFUs, a relatively weak signal. Even with this World Trade Center sample, though, we still might have usable DNA.

While the DNA present wasn't in good shape, some of it might be salvageable. I also knew that there had to be a way to obtain genetic information from samples like that. It was an exercise that took the better part of the next three years to complete.

As the DNA degrades, it approaches the limit of our ability to detect it. When this happens, the specific reactions we use to generate the data are no longer efficient, and the resulting data is unusual: information is missing.

The hallmark of this unusual data is that loci may be missing

FIGURE 3. BADLY DEGRADED DNA

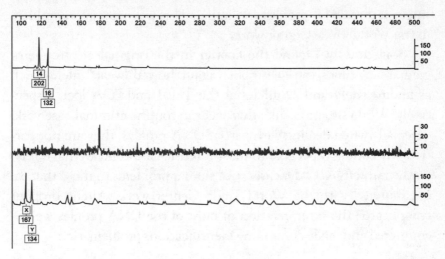

altogether or where there should be two peaks, there is only one. Basically, we are missing data that should be there. We call this phenomenon allelic dropout, which means the instrument did not "call," or report, an allele (a peak). Sometimes we can inspect the electropherogram and find a weak peak that had not been reported. Sometimes the peak is missing altogether.

Consider the following table. Assume that World Trade Center samples DM 1 and DM 2 were found in September 2001. The DNA in these samples appears to be in fairly good shape, and we have complete STR profiles. Now assume that World Trade Center sample DM 3 wasn't recovered until March 2002 at the Staten Island landfill. The DNA profile for DM 3 is missing data: CSF, VWA, and D21S211 are blank. Obviously, this sample has DNA that is significantly degraded.

Compare DM 1 and DM 2 against DM 3. At DM 3, TH01 is missing the 7 allele and FGA is missing the 22 allele. The other alleles at each locus match up with DM 1 and DM 2. The interpretation of this data can get tricky.

We might conclude that DM 1 and DM 2 are not from the same person as DM 3. This might be a possibility, but before concluding that, we have to consider the possibility of allelic dropout, especially since all three STR profiles are similar. This was a common problem in the World Trade Center work.

Sometimes we found the answer in the original electropherogram. Many times, the electropherogram showed "weak" alleles, such as finding the 7 and 22 alleles at the TH01 and FGA loci, respectively. While situations like this occur in routine criminal casework, especially when dealing with partial DNA profiles, they are not particularly common because in most forensic casework, we have relatively fresh DNA. Older cases pose similar problems to those that we encountered with the World Trade Center work. Allelic dropout complicated the interpretation of most of the DNA profiles we encountered and made confirming identifications problematic.

TABLE 4. ALLELIC DROPOUT IN DEGRADED WORLD TRADE CENTER DNA

LOCUS	DM 1 (BONE)	DM 2 (TISSUE)	DMA 3 (BONE)
D2S1358	14, 16	14, 16	14, 16
D16S539	11, 12	11	11, 12
Amelogenin	X, X	X, X	X, X
TH01	6, 7	6, 7	6, 6
TPOX	6, 8	6, 8	6, 8
CSF	11, 11	11, 11	no Signal
D7S820	8, 8	8, 8	8, 8
VWA	17, 18	17, 18	no Signal
FGA	22, 23	22, 23	23, 23
D8S1179	12, 12	12, 12	12, 12
D21S211	27, 28	27, 28	no Signal

During September 2001, my laboratory STR typed the first approximately nine hundred World Trade Center remains accessioned into the laboratory. The first batches gave good results, but by the third week in September, many mimicked the situations illustrated above.

In our Phase I testing, more than 60 percent of the World Trade Center remains gave either partial STR DNA profiles or no profiles. Those remains having partial STR profiles required a different approach, and I began wondering whether there was another way to resurrect the STR data.

7 THE MOST CRITICAL OF TOOLS

In September 2001, the hard fact was that even if we had DNA profiles from all the DMs and all the personal effects and all the kinship swabs, we were still not capable of making even one identification. We had to compare the DNA profiles from family samples with those from the World Trade Center remains. Then we had to align those that matched either directly or indirectly using some as yet unavailable direct-matching or kinship-screening procedure and calculate the probability that we had the proper identification. Finally, we had to assign the name to the DM.

By the end of September, my lab had produced approximately 280 unique STR DNA profiles from World Trade Center remains, but no identifications. Using a crude spreadsheet, we could line up STR profiles and see which remains came from the same person. That is, these were remains having the same DNA profile. This is what Mecki Prinz and I would do for the first 900 STR profiles. Of these 900 STR profiles, we had approximately 280 different individuals—unique profiles—but could not put a name to any of them. However, using a crude spreadsheet without advanced programming was not an appropriate method for making matches. We needed software specifically designed to handle STR data for mass-fatality events. This software did not exist.

Karen Dooling was my lab's CODIS manager. Actually, she had two CODIS responsibilities. She ensured that DNA profiles obtained from regular casework were entered into the system correctly, and she verified matches the system found. She also managed the NYPD backlog casework. It was a huge responsibility.

Karen started in my laboratory in 1994 as a Hofstra University graduate student working on her master's degree in molecular biology. Eventually she took a full-time position as a criminalist, left to take a position in another state agency, and then returned after a year to become an assistant director. She stayed with us, working on the World Trade Center effort until December 2001, when she left to work for the Nassau County Medical Examiner's Office. Her leaving was a blow.

Petite and perky, her ponytail bobbing and swaying as she briskly walked through the lab, Karen is a bright and insightful scientist. I can still see her at her wedding in 1996, scowling at a group of us who traded the warm reception hall for a freezing parking lot where we could listen to the final innings of game six of the World Series.

Karen's CODIS responsibility expanded dramatically during the early World Trade Center DNA effort. With no significant software choices, we had to use CODIS to make direct matches of DMs to personal effects. Karen became the lab's intermediary between the OCME, the FBI, and Science Applications International Corporation, the FBI contract company that authored CODIS.

On September 12, my deputy director, Howard Baum, called Dr. Barry Brown, then the CODIS manager at the FBI, and inquired about the availability of CODIS for the World Trade Center work. Howard did not want the World Trade Center data interfaced with the FBI's nationwide DNA network. I agreed. We both felt it would not be appropriate for the DNA profiles from the remains and family samples to reside in the same network with profiles from the crime scenes of rapes, homicides, and burglaries. Neither of us wanted the perception that the World Trade Center DNA profiles could be searched against those profiles in the national CODIS database. Howard asked for a stand-alone network, one dedicated to the World Trade Center and connected directly to Albany.

Karen shouldered the burden of working with our FBI contact Barry Brown and Science Applications International Corporation. Science Applications International Corporation told her that we could not use our version of CODIS to store the family STR data. It could handle only the DMs. But for the Trade Center work to be successful, the STR profiles from DMs, family samples, and personal effects had to reside in the same database. We needed to be able to search one group against the other electronically. Otherwise we would never make all the identifications. We needed a major CODIS upgrade.

Later on September 12, Mecki Prinz also spoke to Barry Brown. Her e-mail to me said, in part, that Barry expected CODIS to be ready for us in about a week and that Science Applications International Corporation was working overtime. The CODIS upgrade would have an index of human remains and an index of relatives. A statistical feature would be added later for us to calculate kinship probabilities. I accepted what the FBI was doing at face value. Given the magnitude of the World Trade Center work, a week seemed reasonable, but it took much longer.

Then Karen spoke with the FBI on September 14 and learned that our access to the data in Albany would not be over a T1 line. Instead, we would have to use pcAnywhere. This meant the World Trade Center CODIS network connection between Albany and New York City would be molasses slow. I pressed for a T1 line, but that would not be in place until later in 2002. Even then, it did not support CODIS.

I thought there might be a silver lining. Karen had just gotten off the phone with the FBI, and they would be shipping the CODIS upgrade overnight. While the waiting for the upgrade felt like an eternity, in reality, it had been only a few days. But once again I had mistakenly raised my hopes, expecting progress, only to have my spirits dashed. I was rapidly learning that a promise did not translate into a deliverable. Apparently, getting the upgrade code into CODIS was not a trivial matter. The FBI would not install it until later in October.

News from the FBI was always upbeat followed by disappointment. In hindsight, perhaps I should not have been so impatient. The bulk of the samples had not yet been analyzed and the family samples had not even started. Still, I felt the FBI could have been more supportive.

(In February 2004 at the Annual American Academy of Forensic Sciences conference in Dallas, I would learn that Science Applications International Corporation had done additional programming on CODIS using their own money, which, I understand, would have helped us through those initial difficult days. However, the FBI had refused to permit them to contact us to offer their assistance.)

The CODIS upgrade finally arrived, and we named it WTC CODIS. Now we could store the STR DNA data in one of two CODIS indexes: relatives of missing persons and unidentified human remains, which also had personal-effects profiles.

The relatives of the missing persons index in WTC CODIS held DNA profiles from samples taken from relatives of missing persons. These had specific codes: biological mother (BM), biological father (BF), biological son (BS), biological daughter (BD), biological full brother/sister (BU), biological half brother/sister (BH), other (OT)—a catchall category, which might be a maternal or paternal relative, such as a spouse, depending on information provided on a DNA identification report form. A spouse could also be a mother, but came into the laboratory labeled as "spouse." Knowing this enabled us to perform traditional parentage calculations based on the family tree. Although we would have liked additional designations, we used these codes to designate family samples for all of the World Trade Center DNA testing.

Here's how the system worked in the beginning.

As I've explained, the STR data went from Myriad to the New York State Police in Albany on CDs. Peter Wistort, CODIS manager for the state police, and his staff examined the data, performed an error check, then loaded it onto the WTC CODIS server. He ran the matching algorithm and came up with a list of possible matches. Again, these were direct matches, not kinship matches.

Karen announced our first DNA matches on 10/12. Her excitement rang as clear as a bell.

A search was done today at [the] state laboratory. They received 78 unidentified remains profiles back from Myriad. They have also received 103 profiles back from personal items. In addition, there are 113 known exemplars from firefighters (obtained from a bone marrow donation program) that have been profiled by the state police lab and entered into the system.

We received two hits/matches. Two unidentified remains samples matched two toothbrushes. These two were previously identified by OCME through other means. The DNA matches confirm their identity.   ·

For the entire laboratory that worked so hard to produce all the original in house profiles, those profiles are invaluable for Quality Control. They serve as a confirmation to ensure there are no quality problems with the unidentified remains samples being returned from Myriad; this is critical in their initial stages of this project. They were used to confirm the profiles in these first two matches. So thank you all [for] your hard work. We are on our way!

These identifications were direct matches; STR profiles from DMs directly matching personal effects. However, because of the way CODIS made matches, based on high-, medium-, and low-stringency matching parameters, where the stringency correlated to the number of loci allowed to match, Howard Baum and I believed it would create a mountain of unnecessary work as the volume of DM and personal effects data increased.

Peter Wistort confirmed our fears. On October 26, he reported new potential matches—emphasis on the word *potential*. We had

507 total DMs (401 with full profiles and 105 with partial profiles; CODIS did not accept DNA profiles with zero data), 592 from personal effects, 113 samples from firefighters who had donated to a bone marrow donor program, 2,646 family/kin samples. We had 3,857 profiles in World Trade Center CODIS. Peter searched for matches and came up with 1,112 candidates!

Now the work began. CODIS did not print out matches in an easily retrievable format. Karen and her group had to find the samples that matched manually, an enormous task that took weeks. This meant working through paperwork and then creating match groups on a sheet of paper. The enormity of her problem stared me down. At this rate, we would be spending the rest of our lives trying to find identifications.

Karen doesn't know this, but I once had a nightmare of her living at the OCME. Her husband Mike was banging on the door trying desperately to grab her attention, but she was sitting on the floor of the conference room sorting through CODIS match lists. Stacks of candidate match sheets surrounded her, ripped-up and wadded-up paper was strewn around, used color highlighters had been tossed in a corner, her ponytail stuck straight up in the air as though she had poked her finger into an electrical socket.

The week after September 11, I was working at my desk when I noticed a bag sitting on the table in the small conference room adjacent to my office (a glass partition separated my office and the conference room). I peeked into the bag and happily found a treasure trove of individually wrapped brownies: my introduction to Howard Cash. Howard would prove to be one of the World Trade Center families' greatest allies and one of the most indispensable contributors, yet one of its most enigmatic personalities.

Pat Buffolino had known about Gene Codes's commercial software, Sequencher, arguably the most widely used DNA sequence-matching software in the industry. He contacted Howard, the company's founder and president, about obtaining the software for our World Trade Center mtDNA work (at that time I was still trying to figure out whether we would be doing any mtDNA sequencing in-house). Howard sent the brownies to the lab as a gift. His September 19 note to Pat said that when his engineers and quality-assurance team put in unusually long hours, their fuel of choice was brownies from Zingerman's Deli. He hoped our team didn't get too worn out over the next few weeks and months.

I had never met Howard Cash, except through a couple of excellent brownies. Truthfully, I wasn't sure I wanted to. Howard's company had written software to handle DNA sequences, but Pat's interest was specifically mtDNA. Mitotyping was a long way off in the grand scheme of my thinking. I believed I had more important things to occupy my time. Pat had invited him, however, so I felt obliged to at least meet him and listen to what he had to say.

Howard is an interesting character, the consummate traveler. Sometimes he just shows up, almost everywhere, often seemingly uninvited. Three years after September 11, we saw him on TV during the September 11 investigation. From that time, I started calling him Zelig, after the Woody Allen movie. When I mentioned it to Howard, he said, "Zelig by invitation." Still, it's difficult to explain what kind of man he really is. Once he pointed out that I was his first "boss" in fourteen years. He and I know the truth: he had a contract with the city. So while, technically, I might have been his "boss," it didn't take long to learn that Howard really had no boss and that he followed the beat of his own drum, which, frustratingly, was often different from mine.

Physically, Howard is a large man; though not particularly tall, he is portly. His protruding jaw, a family trait, imparts its own special speech characteristics. He's an interesting blend, combining a strong sense of independence and self-confidence spiced with a healthy desire to be recognized, liked, and admired. Certainly one of his more appealing traits is a huge heart and exceedingly strong compassion for the families of the World Trade Center victims. Many times, he and I sat in my office and discussed the tragedy and its impact on us emotionally. Many times we've looked at each other in silence, tacitly acknowledging each other's emotions.

My first conversation with Howard was over the phone on September 16. At first, I was a skeptical and reluctant listener. However, Pat believed Gene Codes had something to offer, so when Howard asked if he could bring a small group to the OCME, my head was saying no, but my mouth agreed.

We met on Saturday, September 28, though earlier that morning, I chided myself for even scheduling the meeting, and I thought about breaking the date. I'm glad I didn't. Howard brought several people with him: Mike Hennessey, who worked to almost the pause; Debra Cash, Howard's sister; Dr. Judy Nolan; and David Feldt. At Howard's request, I outlined the flow of samples, remains, and informatics—the flow of information and data—both inside my laboratory and within the OCME as I understood them.

David Feldt impressed immediately. He opened my mind with thoughts about things I had not heard before. I felt like we clicked. Though I would meet him only one more time, he set my thinking in the proper direction.

David's description of metadata and middleware software struck a chord. I had never heard of metadata or middleware, and it took me several minutes to figure out what the heck he was talking about. But he was adamant that it would become important in the DNA identification process. Until that meeting, I firmly believed that DNA was the best way to make identifications. I did not completely appreciate how non-DNA data, beyond the traditional identification modalities like medical anomalies, personal effects, dental records, and fingerprints, could help make DNA identifications.

Middleware software was also a new term, and it took a while before I understood its importance. It would be more than a year and a half before I asked Gene Codes Forensics to program a mechanism to use middleware to guide me toward new identifications.

Gene Codes is a molecular biology software company. After our Saturday meeting, I did not commit to them to write the code for what would become the software we would eventually use the most for the World Trade Center DNA effort. I was still waiting for the FBI to step up to the plate. I suppose I was misguided by loyalty to my traditional law enforcement roots. Privately, I was praying the FBI would commission Science Applications International Corporation to write a customized CODIS upgrade.

I should've known better. My personal dealings with the FBI over the years had always left me wanting. And though I secretly prayed they'd do the job, I had the nagging doubt that they either could not or, through some bizarre bureaucratic obstinacy, would not.

On the day I met with Howard Cash, I still had no software tool available to help, and I needed to convene a group of experts. I needed to know what was available to me.

I met with the experts and organizations I thought might help solve this critical problem. There was one critical truth: without the appropriate software to help analyze the DNA data, I was lost. The families were lost. I might as well have packed my bags and left town. I asked Howard Cash to attend the October 3 "summit" meeting.

Dr. Charles Brenner's business card reads, "Aphorisms, Inferences, and Conclusions from Thin Air." He's a unique individual, a man whom you must treasure for who he is. In his late fifties, Charles is tall—truthfully, most people are taller than I am—and thin. He wears a fedora and occasionally steadies himself with a cane. A self-styled freelance consultant, Charles fancies himself a forensic mathematician and population geneticist. He also professes being a computer guru, having worked with them since 1959. Unquestionably, his contribution to the World Trade Center DNA effort was monumental.

Charles is the author of a DNA parentage software package, DNAView, an early version of which my laboratory had been using for years. At the time, it was the most sophisticated, commercially available parentage/kinship analysis program available. Although my laboratory was not a New York State Department of Health–certified paternity testing facility, we did conduct forensic paternity testing in those instances when we needed to establish the identity of a body or to prove that an arrested man was the father of a child born in the aftermath of a sexual assault.

DNAView is DOS-based, a dinosaur in a world captured by Windows and budding Linux operating systems. I've not subtly suggested to Charles that he upgrade DNAView to make it compatible with modern operating systems. I'd guess he simply needed the funding. Three years later, I believe this was happening in conjunction with a major software company.

DNAView is a hodgepodge of add-ons, as Charles continually added features as needed. The program is clunky, buggy, nonintuitive, and frustrating. It's also the best at what it does. Once I had DNAViews in my hands, I sat alone at my computer many mornings, ferreting my way around its idiosyncratic menus willing it to do what I wanted. If it were not for the fact that without DNAView a large percentage of families would never have their loved ones returned, I might have tossed it into a virtual circular file.

Although Charles had visited my laboratory several times, and we had an annual contract with him to upgrade DNAView, my personal contact with him before the World Trade Center attacks was minimal. My first real encounter with him was at the summit meeting in October, where he illustrated the problems we faced in identifying such a large number of people. In an understatement, he said, "It isn't a trivial task."

My second glimpse of his personality occurred at the first Kinship and Data Analysis Panel in October. I was sitting beside him listening to one of the panel scientists make an abstract point. Charles leaned over and said, "I thought I invented that."

I replied, "I don't doubt it. Maybe you should sue."

Charles looked at me for a long moment, as if he were seriously considering the remark. Charles is a quietly outspoken man who has incredible faith in his own brilliance and opinions. I do believe he lives on the fringe of brilliance.

On September 11, Howard Baum asked me if he should contact

Charles. I didn't know who else to call. Benoit Leclair was a choice because of his work with the Royal Canadian Mounted Police in the Swissair crash. But Charles was also a logical choice because of DNAView, though I believed we needed more than what was available in DNAView. We needed a parentage screen of thousands of DMs compared against thousands of kinship samples. At the time, DNAView did not have that capability, as it handled only one sample at a time.

Charles's Web site has a World Trade Center Disaster Identification Diary. On September 12, he mentions receiving an e-mail from Howard Baum. He writes, "The OCME has been using the kinship module of DNAView for several years, and it is already well established as a tool for disaster body identification. I shouldn't have needed Howard to remind me. His message was brief. He wrote, 'We need help coping with the mass disaster in New York City.'"

Typically, Charles believed he had more to offer than just his kinship analysis program. He speculated correctly that there would be a lot of genetic data to manipulate, the nature of which couldn't be predicted in advance.

He continued, "As one who has worked with computers since 1959, earned a doctorate in mathematics, and done dozens of practical or research projects involving DNA-relationship ideas and computations, I figure I am uniquely prepared to perform whatever manipulations and analysis [that] might be necessary to wring information from the data."

Charles, I hope, would now readily confess that the kinship module of DNAView needed serious tweaking before it was ready to handle the World Trade Center kinship exercise.

Swissair Flight III crashed off the coast of Nova Scotia with 229 aboard. While the Royal Canadian Mounted Police assumed the grim task of identifying the missing, the credibility of these identifications became the responsibility of one man: Dr. Benoit Leclair.

An extremely proud man, slim and of medium height, his long

French face, affable smile, and intense, piercing blue eyes define him to a T. Benoit is the only person who worked on the World Trade Center DNA effort, other than civil servants, who did not have a contractual agreement with the city. The company he worked for, Myriad Genetics Laboratories, was under contract to the New York State Police and was the first private forensic laboratory I employed to STR type World Trade Center tissue extracts. Aside from his Myriad salary, Benoit was never paid for his efforts, even though he did substantial work on his own time.

He certainly deserved to be paid because he worked tirelessly, spending weekends sequestered from his family, continually processing data, and writing and rewriting code to update his DNA program, MDKAP, to handle the constantly changing nomenclature and DNA tests. I hope his family is proud of his accomplishment. I know the World Trade Center families are eternally grateful.

Benoit had taken Excel to its logical limits by adapting its programming language into a DNA mass-disaster body identification tool, evolving it into the program that he calls MDKAP (Mass Disaster Kinship Analysis Program), which is available commercially under the name of Bloodhound.

Conceptually, his approach was similar to though significantly more sophisticated than the FBI's plan for CODIS. Also, Benoit's program differed substantially in principle from Charles's DNAView. On September 11, however, these differences did not matter. I simply wanted to know whether it would help. Because of the magnitude of the World Trade Center disaster compared with the Swissair crash, I had my reservations.

As it turns out, I had bureaucratic problems to solve before I could set eyes on the program, so understanding how Benoit's software might help and having it in-house turned out to be two different things. I was not privy to all the behind-the-scenes maneuvering, but getting a copy proved frustrating. Anecdotally, there were proprietary issues with the Royal Canadian Mounted Police, who owned the software, and then there was some mysterious issue about the Swissair data, which I did not want and really didn't care about. Somehow, not surprisingly, the FBI was involved. I have no idea why.

It took a while, but eventually Benoit made plans to visit New York. However, an e-mail from Howard Baum on 9/25 said, in part, that Benoit has not been able to coordinate with the FBI, and that they might ask him to postpone his trip to New York. There was something about Benoit verifying the FBI software (I suppose CODIS), which led Howard to speculate, "It sounds like the FBI software may be delayed." That was our first hint that the CODIS upgrade would be delayed.

Benoit eventually made it to Albany and the New York State Police and then to us at the OCME. At first glance, MDKAP was confusing. Its elegance becomes apparent only after one learns how to use it. It enabled us to make kinship identifications that DNAView could not.

Mark Dale and I agreed to have a full-time project manager assist the running of the daily World Trade Center operation. I needed someone who could interface between the New York State Police and the OCME. The idea was Mark's.

The World Trade Center work was consuming a huge amount of Barry Duceman's resources, and Mark was spending a significant proportion of his time, too. I am guessing, but I suppose he must have had tremendous pressure to return to managing the Forensic Investigation Center full-time. Barry's laboratory had its own caseload. Clearly, the World Trade Center effort was the OCME's responsibility.

I was completely overwhelmed and continually worried that I would lose track amid the turmoil. I often felt like I was supporting a house of cards teetering on a cliff overlooking the ocean. One mistake and it would tumble into the boiling surf, taking me with it. Also, having time alone to collect my thoughts would have been a welcome respite. So the suggestion of a project manager was appealing. I also liked the thought of having someone with whom to work, someone who could field my ideas and give unbiased feedback.

Steve Niezgoda came to the OCME in early December 2001. It took only a few days before I was feeling as comfortable with him as I have with anyone.

After I got to know him better, I would tease him about most everything from his taste in beer to his inability to hold liquor. Steve's a husky guy and could easily pound me into the ground if he chose to, but he's mild mannered, has a quick smile, and an easygoing personality.

My only reservation was knowing that Steve had worked for the FBI and had a huge responsibility with CODIS; his name is associated with early publications about the FBI's crowning DNA achievement. I admit my bias was rooted in my disappointing FBI experience at the beginning of the World Trade Center effort. None of that was Steve's fault or CODIS's. But Steve was intimately familiar with CODIS's strengths and weaknesses, and I believed this would be a bonus for the World Trade Center families.

Leaving the FBI must have been a hard decision for him, but it turned out to be a huge win for me, the World Trade Center DNA identification effort, and the families.

Once on board, Steve quickly established a close working relationship with Peter Wistort at the state police in Albany. I needed to know that the data Peter input into World Trade Center CODIS was of good quality. In order to keep Peter from drowning in the data, Steve wrote a script that allowed Peter and his staff to quickly evaluate the data. It was a huge help because it provided an electronic mechanism to check the STR data coming from Myriad and, later, from Bode and my laboratory.

I watched Steve closely for several weeks. He worked well with my staff and coordinated with the New York State Police scientists in Albany. I decided he should be the permanent liaison between the two agencies. His knowledge of software, databases, and CODIS, and his experience as a project manager—skills I barely possess—made him the perfect candidate.

In mid-December, I needed to change the World Trade Center management structure. Although I had the responsibility, practically,

Howard Baum and I had been sharing the role, and it was rapidly becoming an impossible relationship. The World Trade Center work needed one person to be in charge, and when Howard and I were making contradictory decisions on the same issues, I knew a change had to happen. I could not afford for anyone to perceive us as having a conflict. It was potentially embarrassing and, with media scrutiny escalating, I needed a single spokesperson for the DNA work.

With Steve on board I asked Howard to concentrate more on the daily casework, which was suffering from a lack of technical leadership, and I wanted Howard to reassume his role as the lab's technical leader.

Understandably, Howard was far from happy, but he agreed. In truth, I did not remove him completely from the World Trade Center work. He continued to chair the Kinship and Data Analysis Panel mtDNA and software committees. Later, he and I reviewed the validation data for new technologies we developed.

There was a hitch in making Steve the project manager. Steve was a National Institute of Justice contractor, and his contract would not allow it. He had been brought on board to help with CODIS and to help solve problems associated with implementing World Trade Center CODIS, which he did admirably. So I had to use him in a way that was acceptable to the National Institute of Justice. Steve became my silent, unofficial World Trade Center project manager. Actually, he did both. He worked ostensibly under his National Institute of Justice contract while working with me on the World Trade Center effort.

His work schedule was tough. He commuted to New York from Manassas, Virginia, three days a week. As the unofficial go-between for the OCME and the New York State Police, he'd be in either Albany or the city. Most of the time, he was in New York City. He coordinated the identification activities of the second-floor World Trade Center DNA identification unit. I never had to ask if he was there. I simply had to look at his desk for the telltale signs: a partially empty can of Diet Coke and a small bag of potato chips.

I quickly learned that Steve is a terrific manager. He had a handle on how we were transferring samples among laboratories, and he understood my insane desire to know which laboratory analyzed which sample using which test. I believed this was important information for anyone examining what we did in the future. It turned out to be a nightmare nomenclature problem, but Steve was on it.

After Steve took the day-to-day reins in late December, I had more time to concentrate on the more global issues and found myself spending more time in the identification unit in the early morning. For the approximately three months he helped to manage the daily grind, I felt more confident we were getting a grip on the work. He kept a lid on the effort and streamlined several operations. He organized the identification team and carefully monitored all CODIS downloads—we called them dumps—and helped me whenever I needed him.

Early on, Steve instituted a series of weekly logistics meetings. I was always the first speaker on the agenda. Five minutes before the meeting, Steve came into my office and handed me a piece of paper— the agenda. I am sure he secretly relished watching my surprise when I had to hustle to find the unexpected agenda items.

On December 21, my mother-in-law suffered the first of two hemorrhagic strokes. My wife Fran and I flew to Florida to be with her. I stayed a week, but Fran stayed until February, when she brought her mother to New Jersey. While I was in Florida, Steve ran the World Trade Center operation and kept me abreast of what was happening.

When I returned in December and was living alone, Steve and I spent hours talking well into the evening over dinner and beer. This was an important time for us because it cemented our working and personal relationships. We talked openly about the World Trade Center work, gaining respect and trust for each other. Once, I confessed we'd be lucky to identify 50 percent of those who died.

Since Steve is such an affable person, it was a surprise to find him embroiled in a personality conflict. However, unknown to me, one was brewing, one that could affect the entire World Trade Center DNA effort.

8 THE SUMMIT MEETING

September 30, 2001

Missing Identified: 221

DNA Identifications: 0

Personal Effects at New York State Police: 153

Remains Received: 4,789

The October 3, 2001, headline in the *Wall Street Journal* read: "Summit Called to Map Strategy on Victims' DNA."

At the time, describing the meeting as a "summit" wasn't how I thought of the group of scientists I asked to meet with me in New York. It could have more appropriately been titled, "OCME Scientist Desperate for Help." I needed expertise in the World Trade Center fold.

In hindsight, though, the meeting might have been a summit because the scientists who attended became an integral part of the World Trade Center DNA effort. This group's expertise, experience, and connections could lead us to the people or organizations who had access to the capability to perform a number of diverse tasks. At the time, my laboratory did not have the capability to identify those who died. But I thought we could handle the DNA testing part by partnering with the New York State Police. We had established a workable mechanism to ensure that DNA typing would be done on both World Trade Center DMs and the family samples. But that was only half the job, and lacking the ability to do the other half—the actual identification part—evoked a helpless feeling.

I had no way to convert DNA test results into identifications. It was disturbing because it meant we could fail, and with Chuck Hirsch, the mayor, the New York City Fire Department, the New York City Police Department, and the media watching with high expectations, I felt the pressure to turn out identifications quickly. Thankfully, at this stage, the families had not yet tuned in to DNA and its importance in identifying their loved ones. Had they understood, I am certain the pressure would have been intolerable.

What was more unsettling—and I was just beginning to realize it—was that nothing on the planet existed to do this job properly. I needed a software solution as much as I need my arms. I had to be able to analyze DNA profiles obtained from samples collected at the World Trade Center site and match them to families. DNA data would be streaming into the laboratory, and I had to be ready to use it.

In mass disasters, identifications are made using a variety of forensic techniques. Dental records and fingerprints of the missing are the most commonly employed. Additionally, metadata—such as an employment ID card found inside the wallet from a pair of pants on a headless torso—can also provide important clues, though relying on this kind of information without supporting evidence might be problematic.

Using DNA for identification purposes in mass fatalities was relatively new. The underlying technology developed in the late 1980s by Alex Jefferies at the University of Leicester in England was not used extensively for mass-disaster identifications because the technology, called DNA Fingerprinting at the time, was both tedious and time consuming. It wasn't until the crash of TWA Flight 800, after a wing fuel tank exploded in midair off the coast of Long Island, that STR DNA analysis was used to identify victims of a mass disaster.

Manual DNA matching techniques using spreadsheets are common and perhaps even appropriate in airline crashes, where there is a limited and known number of casualties, but they are inappropriate for mass fatalities the size of the World Trade Center disaster. I was expecting thousands of DMs, each of which had to be analyzed and tracked. There would also be thousands of family samples that had to be compared to these DMs. Only software designed specifically for that purpose would be effective and efficient.

Minimally, the software had to perform direct-matching chores efficiently. It had to line up matching DNA profiles quickly, so we could ascertain which disaster samples, or DMs, matched the personal effects from the missing. Also, grouping fragmented remains that belonged to a single person, even if a name was not known, was another task the software had to perform. This we called pieces-to-pieces matching or, more technically, repatriation of the remains.

That was only the direct-matching part of the DNA identification puzzle. The software also had to perform kinship analysis, where a family's DNA—that is, its genetic structure—could be matched to a DM, as in a sophisticated paternity test. All I had at that moment was CODIS, which had not been designed for either purpose.

By the summit meeting, my laboratory was pumping out DNA profiles on DMs, and so was Myriad for the family samples. We had completed DNA analysis on more than 900 DMs, which yielded nearly 280 unique profiles. This meant that DNA could potentially identify almost 280 of the missing people. But without the right software, I could not name them.

Now I had the experts in the same room, and it was showtime. My goal was to come away from the meeting with a plan of action. I wanted them to tell me how I was going to solve this problem.

These summit experts, either singly or representing their organizations, worked with us from that meeting on. They included Dr. Bruce Budowle, who worked in the research division of the FBI and had for years spearheaded many of the FBI's biological initiatives. At crucial times over the next two years, Bruce was a lone supporter of my new technology initiatives. Dr. Barry Brown was the FBI's CODIS manger. Dr. Joe DiZinno was the assistant director of the FBI laboratory. Howard Cash was the founder and president of Gene Codes Forensics. Rhonda Roby was a scientist with Applied Biosystems, a Celera Genomics sister company, who supervised Soaring Eagles, the

Celera Genomics code for its World Trade Center mitochondrial DNA work. Dr. Tim Stockwell and Dr. Gene Meyers were scientists at Celera Genomics. Dr. Barry Duceman and Mark Dale were from the New York State Police. Dr. Benoit Leclair was a scientist at Myriad Genetics and the author of MDKAP, a kinship and direct-matching software program we were considering. Dr. Charles Brenner was the author of DNAView, one of the software programs we were considering; he was also an OCME consultant. Dr. Lisa Forman was the director of research programs for the National Institute of Justice and also the architect of the Kinship and Data Analysis Panel.

The meeting lasted most of the day. I had purposely designed a loose agenda so that the group could explore alternative approaches for sorting through the mass of anticipated data. In the morning, each participant gave a short presentation with respect to making the necessary victim-to-reference matches. The afternoon found us brainstorming, probably a bit too much, so we ended the day by establishing a software panel that Howard Baum would chair.

Charles Brenner presented DNAView, a program we had been using in-house for parentage analysis. As always, his presentation had an interesting bent because he leaned toward mathematical modeling to emphasize many of his points. True to form, Charles's Web site offered this: ". . . once I am able to get my hands on the data, I will quite quickly be able to produce the tentative identifications by myself." I chuckled when I read that because it was typically Charles, who now, I hope, would admit it would be a daunting undertaking, even for him.

Howard Cash responded with obviously a tongue-in-cheek, good-natured rib spiced with a hint of sarcasm: "Surely, Charles, even your work can stand a second opinion."

Charles thought a moment before replying, "You have a fair point."

Benoit showed us how he had used an Excel-based program (eventually named MDKAP and now marketed under the name Bloodhound) to make kinship matches in the Swissair crash. This was the second time someone had shown me Benoit's program. Again, I was impressed. Again, I found it difficult to follow.

The FBI's Dr. Barry Brown and Dr. Joe DiZinno explained how CODIS might help. They proposed using CODIS to do what is known as a pairwise comparison of alleles. While this was similar to Benoit Leclair's MDKAP, CODIS would give us only an unsorted list of potential matches. Benoit listed candidate matches according to the ones most likely to be correct, along with statistical probabilities. After listening to the FBI's idea, I thought about the extra work Karen Dooling had to do in making simple direct matches for our routine criminal work. My take-home lesson for the day was that CODIS was not ready for kinship analysis. Howard Baum also had his doubts. We discussed using CODIS for kinship analysis and agreed that the FBI's approach would give us a Pandora's box of false matches.

After the day ended, I had exactly what I started with: nothing. Well, that's not precisely true. I had confirmed what I suspected: nothing existed that could do the job. Certainly, CODIS could do direct matching, rudimentary as it would be, but I knew that already. Benoit's program, MDKAP, could not handle multiple DNA profiles searched against multiple DNA profiles, and DNAView was not ready for a project this size.

I left the meeting with a bad feeling. I had to update Chuck Hirsch, and I was not looking forward to handing him such bad news. The newspapers would be calling and that would not be pleasant. It was tremendously depressing.

Although I stubbornly, and perhaps naively, harbored hopes the FBI would upgrade CODIS to meet our requirements, I increasingly felt compelled to have a second iron in the fire.

When I left the summit meeting, I was torn between CODIS and jettisoning it for an entirely new software program. By the time I walked back into my office, I had made a decision, which I kept private. It would be the most important World Trade Center decision I would make.

• • •

While I wrestled with software issues, my laboratory continued to pump out DNA profiles on tissue DMs, the final number at this early stage being 943. But by the end of September, we had received 4,789 DMs. The New York State Police had 2,770 case files from families but had completed cataloging only 112 bloodstains, 52 family swabs, and 89 prepared bloodstain cards. Myriad had not yet received DNA extracts from tissue DMs.

Getting tissue extracts into Myiad's hands turned out to be a struggle. The first 3,000, which my laboratory had extracted manually, were stored in small, individual 1.5-milliliter conical plastic tubes, microcentrifuge tubes. Myriad, however, preferred microtiter plates (plastic plates that held 96 samples) instead of individual tubes because they fit nicely into their high-throughput format. This meant my staff had to transfer the tissue DNA extracts from individual tubes into the microtiter plates. This was a huge job because it had to be done carefully in order to keep the DM extracts straight.

In getting these extracts to Myriad, we also ran into unexpected problems. Mecki sent Myriad trial microtiter plates. We went through a period of sending trial samples back and forth to ensure that Myriad's software could read our bar-code labels. The process was one of setting both laboratories on the same page, and we had to do it with all of our contract vendors. In one instance, Mecki sent samples out on a Friday. FedEx guaranteed a Saturday delivery. Well, Saturday came and went, and Myriad had no samples. They didn't arrive until Monday. We had to retrieve the samples and then reextract the original DMs. After that, we never trusted a delivery company's promise again. No DM extracts ever left the OCME on a Friday after that or if there was even a hint of a possible delivery problem.

9 AN ALTERNATE TEST

Managing the World Trade Center was not my only fall 2001 distraction. The city's Office of Management and Budget had me buried in the second phase of a value engineering study. Value engineering is the term for a process whereby the city has a second group of engineers reexamine plans for new construction projects. This was the second of these, the first of which had taken place earlier that spring.

We had received mayoral approval for a new forensic biology building. For me, a lowly civil servant, this was a dream come true. I wanted this laboratory to be the city's crown jewel of forensic science, and I set my sights on developing the most innovative, forward-thinking forensic entity in the country. We had the talent and, I hoped, the resources to make it happen. It was very exciting.

When it comes to forensic science, law enforcement has not historically been especially innovative. I regarded our new forensic biology building as a chance to change that and to interject my philosophy into a city that, in my experience, had a spotty forensic track record. I wanted my colleagues to stand up and notice how far New York had come. I wanted those who for years had snickered privately at New York's forensic ineptness to acknowledge that we had taken a leadership role.

Chuck Hirsch always believed that the DNA lab's stellar track record would create its own recognition, and that the city could not ignore our work forever. But when we were given the opportunity to design a new building, I was skeptical. The DNA laboratory had already proven itself an indispensable investigative tool, an important cog in the city's law enforcement machine. I still harbored fears that the NYPD believed the DNA lab was theirs for the taking, which would mean a strict devotion to criminal cases, the routine. The routine stuff really was the bread and butter, the necessary boring stuff. But I believed there was more that could and should be done.

Under an NYPD-controlled system, the chief of detectives would call at 2:00 A.M. and demand I get someone into the lab to do a DNA test on some rape kit. It happened. When a detective, a captain, or an inspector "perceived" a suspect was a "bad guy" or if someone suggested that the suspect "looked like," say, the East Side Rapist, the inane, demand-a-result-approach to science started. Frustrating as such ignorance about good science can be, it's not surprising. They're cops, not scientists. They, too, have a job to do.

Though the building would be constructed as an OCME project with a similar but sometimes completely different agenda than the NYPD, I feared having the NYPD on the planning committee—a necessary evil—would stifle my chance to make this something special. During these meetings, I often wondered whether I could get away with designing something special, something the city really needed, and also fulfill a dream.

Municipal governments have an abysmal track record for designing with vision. Mostly, new construction has today's needs in mind, rhetoric to the contrary. Thankfully, the new DNA building project was different from the get go. Everyone associated with the project, the NYPD included, agreed this building had to have a flexible design so it could adapt to future technology. We hired a progressive laboratory design firm, HERA, in St. Louis.

Rhetoric or not, I embraced the enthusiasm as if it were a mandate. I added features that most municipal government scientists could only dream of. I had a fully staffed training laboratory, a separate, miniature clone of the casework laboratory (a 9/11 afterthought), which would be on emergency power with a BSL-3 capability in the event of a weapons of mass destruction event. There was a research laboratory so that we could evaluate new methods and implement new ideas without impacting casework. I also had a molecular pathology laboratory, which would identify the specific mutation on the DNA that caused someone's death. The plan was to offer genetic counseling to those families and then provide a no-charge genetic analysis to family members so that the families would know who might be at risk for certain diseases or conditions. The OCME would be the first in the nation to offer this type of testing based on autopsy findings. The laboratory offered the first of a planned battery of tests in April 2005. And there was a forensic neurobiology laboratory that would embrace what I believe might be the next important arena of forensic biology.

One day in spring 2001, after I had spent a long day hashing over design details, an Office of Management and Budget manager came in and asked how many of us would like to attend the opening of the genome exhibit at the Museum of Natural History. I wasn't sure if I wanted to. It meant getting home late, which translated into a sluggish brain the next morning. However, my lab was supposed to have an exhibit, so I decided I should go.

It turned out to be a gala affair. The entrance to the museum had huge tables of hors d'oeuvres and wine stations where one could get a strange blue drink served in a laboratory beaker reworked into a drinking vessel. A group of us were walking through the exhibit when Teri Michaud, an Office of Management and Budget staffer and an OCME contact for the new building project, pointed out a man surrounded by several attractive young women. In another venue, he might have been a rock star surrounded by groveling groupies. No rock star this time. He was Dr. Craig Venter, the founder of Celera Genomics, the private company that had sequenced the human genome in direct competition with a public effort led by Dr. Francis Collins of the National Institutes of Health.

In a bold move, Craig had challenged the establishment, claiming he could sequence the human genome in a fraction of the time originally planned. Well, this lit a fire under the Human Genome Consortium, and the race was on. Craig succeeded but incurred the wrath of his governmental colleagues. In the end, science and the world won. Both groups completed the task in a dead heat.

I wanted to meet Craig Venter because I admired his irreverence. I'm not someone who forces his attention on famous people, anyone actually, because I respect their privacy. Also, I'm basically shy. Craig was enjoying—no, relishing—being the center of attention. I studied him for a few minutes, trying to work up the courage to introduce myself. He certainly wouldn't know who I was, but I did represent the largest forensic DNA lab in the country, and I thought meeting him might benefit us sometime in the future.

With Teri goading me, I swallowed hard and approached him. At first, I had trouble forging my way through his entourage, so I stood on the perimeter of his group for what felt like an eternity. When he finally finished his conversation, I stuck out my hand and introduced myself. I was shocked at how easy it was.

Howard Baum, who was with me, and I chatted with Craig for about five minutes. Though I was nervous the entire time, I left feeling good about the experience. He was gracious. As I remember him that night, he seemed like a leprechaun, his dancing blue eyes matching perfectly a vibrant and expressive personality.

I was surprised when Craig called on Wednesday, September 12.

Human cells have two kinds of DNA. The DNA most of us are familiar with is called genomic DNA, which resides inside the cell's nucleus. It comprises the 46 chromosomes that house the DNA we normally think of as being responsible for our genetic inheritance. It's the same DNA scientists use for cloning, like Lucy the sheep and now cats. It is also the major perpetrator of inherited diseases, the basis of our physical appearance, and the mechanism of forensic human identification in criminal and parentage cases. This is the DNA I had to tap for making identifications in our World Trade Center work.

Genomic DNA is a huge, linear molecule structured much like a twisted ladder. The rungs of the ladder are called base pairs, of which there are approximately 3 billion. They contain DNA's four-letter universal code, ACTG, the sequence of which is individually unique, except for identical twins.

With almost none of the Human Genome Project's ballyhoo, a second DNA lurks quietly inside our cells, too. Called mitochondrial DNA (mtDNA), it resides inside mitochondria, the small bacteria-shaped organelles inside a cell's cytoplasm. It is much smaller than genomic DNA and circular in structure, having only 16,569 base pairs. Importantly, mitochondria control the energy requirements of the cells. So heart cells, which require huge amounts of energy to keep beating, need more mitochondria than, say, skin cells, which don't work that hard.

Mitochondrial DNA is special because it is inherited maternally, which means a mother and her children share the same mtDNA. Siblings having the same mother have the same mtDNA. But a father may not have the same mtDNA as his biological children.

There are other important differences between mtDNA and genomic DNA. For example, each mitochondrion has a single copy of mtDNA, just as the nucleus has a single copy of genomic DNA. However, each cell may have multiple mitochondria and thus many copies of mtDNA. The cell, however, has only one copy of genomic DNA because each cell has only one nucleus. Like genomic DNA, though, mutations in the mtDNA sequence may cause disease.

Forensic scientists use mtDNA primarily for body identifications. Because mtDNA is housed inside the mitochondrion and has multiple copies inside each cell, some scientists believe that this, plus its circular structure, makes it hardier than genomic DNA and thus more resistant to deterioration in decomposing tissue. Not surprisingly, medical examiners have become enamored of mtDNA because it is often available when genomic DNA is not.

In that first week after the World Trade Center attacks, Chuck specifically asked if we were planning to do mtDNA typing on all of the DMs. The implication was clear: he wanted it done. Though I answered affirmatively, I had reservations.

Most of the mitochondrial genome is relatively static and doesn't differ greatly among individuals. This is probably true because most of the mitochondrial genome is responsible for providing energy to cells, where continual changing of the mtDNA code could lead to cellular malfunction and death. For body identifications, scientists determine the DNA sequence of only a small region of the mitochondrial genome, called the D-loop, which is anything but static.

Having no known function, the D-loop varies greatly among individuals. So, for body identification purposes, scientists compare the D-loop sequence against a consensus sequence called the Cambridge Reference Sequence. Differences between the two sequences are put into a tabular format called a mitotype, which should match the maternal lineage of the family.

Simply obtaining a mitotype from a DM is not sufficient to make an identification, especially when dealing with a large population of missing people. As I mentioned, mitotypes are not necessarily unique, and many individuals share the same mitotype without being related; approximately 7 percent of all Caucasians have the same D-loop. Additionally, mtDNA sequences can lead to interpretation problems, which are highly technical and outside the scope of this discussion.

Technically, determining the sequence of mtDNA is far from simple. The reigning forensic science paradigm for mtDNA sequencing requires determining the sequence of both strands of the mtDNA—the backbones of the DNA ladder. This is called forward and reverse sequencing. Then, two scientists must examine both sequences and agree. This is simply good science. The mass-fatality paradigm for using mtDNA has always been this: use mtDNA for body identifications only as necessary.

There is a practical reason for this. Most laboratories performing forensic mtDNA sequencing can produce only a few mitotypes each week. For the World Trade Center, where I was expecting thousands of samples, this posed a problem. There were not enough forensic mtDNA sequencing laboratories in the country that could do the work. Nor were there enough forensic scientists who knew mtDNA sequencing well enough to do the necessary reviews.

Eventually I would need mitotypes on disaster samples as well as the maternal lineage of the families. Pat Buffolino had completed our laboratory's validation of mtDNA sequencing and was urging me to do it on DMs. In this instance, validating meant demonstrating that sequencing mtDNA on degraded human remains was reliable.

I guessed we could produce perhaps ten mitotypes weekly, though Pat believed we might do more. Even if he could triple our output, it wasn't nearly enough to carry out Chuck Hirsch's wishes for mtDNA sequencing on all the World Trade Center disaster samples in addition to potentially thousands of family samples. It wasn't looking good. Because of the overwhelming number of DMs we would receive, I assumed that mitotyping DMs would be done only to confirm a possible identification.

No one had ever attempted universal mtDNA sequencing on disaster samples, mainly because the technology simply did not exist to handle that quantity of samples and still have them pass forensic muster. But universal mtDNA sequencing was precisely what I needed.

Craig Venter called just after I had hung up from speaking with Arne Masibay of Promega about robotic systems. I was still in a daze and, now, I had Craig Venter on the phone. He spoke so rapidly I managed to catch only a few phrases at a time. I thought I heard him mention something about speaking to someone in the mayor's office, or was it the governor, or was it some senator? Maybe it was all of them. I couldn't really be certain. I really didn't care.

"We can do one hundred thousand sequences a day," he bragged.

The number kept rattling inside my head. Had I heard him correctly? I remember saying something completely inane: "That's really impressive."

Inside, I was both skeptical and excited.

I rarely warm up easily to people who flaunt their political connections to foster their own end. And I hate having someone bully me. I guess it's my stubborn Irish temperament that rapidly turns sour when I'm backed into a corner. From my perspective, the tenor of the conversation with Craig wasn't going well. I wasn't sure I even believed him.

As I mentioned, most forensic labs produce only a few mitotypes a week. Could Celera actually sequence mtDNA? I had to believe they could. Human Genome Project controversy aside, Celera's scientists had sequenced the human genome. No one doubted that. Had he really said one hundred thousand sequences a day? If he was only 1/100th accurate, it would be a miracle. At that moment, I thought the mass-fatality mtDNA paradigm shifted.

"How many samples?" Craig asked excitedly.

I had no clue. "Maybe as many as one hundred thousand," I said. "But we're not really sure." On day two, I hadn't given much thought to the number of samples we would receive, and I had no way to make an educated guess.

My mind was racing. Could we really use universal mitotyping to identify World Trade Center bodies? Could Celera do it?

10 A REMARKABLE WOMAN

I have been given credit for orchestrating the entire DNA effort, marrying technology and scientists into a cohesive, well-oiled, mass-fatality DNA identification machine. However, to have achieved even a modicum of success, I have relied on managers and scientists, inside and outside of the OCME, who performed specific tasks, each vital for identifying those who perished.

The most visible and those most written about by the print media were the private laboratories: Myriad Genetics Laboratory, the Bode Technology Group, Celera Genomics, and Orchid Cellmark in Dallas. Scientists in these laboratories, under the direction of their managers, performed the DNA testing, some routine and some highly specialized. Each of these laboratories contributed mightily to the World Trade Center work.

Public laboratories, such as my laboratory and the New York State Police lab in Albany, also performed DNA testing, which brought the total number of active DNA laboratories working on this incredibly complex World Trade Center project to six. Another critical group of scientists working inside the OCME evaluated all the DNA data using software supplied by vendors, making the identifications by putting names to DNA profiles from DMs. And then there was Dr. John Butler at the National Institute of Standards and Technology, who did some groundbreaking research. This brought the number of DNA laboratories to seven.

Each of these organizations comprised individual parts of the whole effort, where each individual part had a manager or supervisor with whom I worked closely. Dr. Mitch Holland and his wife, Charity, at Bode, Dr. Bob Giles at Orchid, and Rhonda Roby at Celera were in my ear almost daily, often helping and working with my staff and theirs. These were the most visible groups. One group, a critical one, was not so visible. It was the brainchild of another not-so-visible but very special person.

They say that there is a woman behind every successful man. I've wondered whether this meant a nagging wife or confidante who somehow had the knack of keeping his foot out of his mouth. Certainly, Franklin had Eleanor and Ronnie had Nancy. Though the adage may not always hold true, I believe the premise generally does. Women perceive the world differently than men do. They have an uncanny ability to keep critical issues in perspective and to make sense out of chaos, which is certainly something I needed. Throughout the entire DNA identification effort, I had the extreme good fortune of having several superbly qualified women working with me. For now, one stands out.

Dr. Lisa (pronounced Leeza) Forman, then the director of the Investigative and Forensic Sciences Division at the National Institute of Justice (NIJ), visited New York in late September and asked Mark Dale and me what kind of help we needed.

Lisa has a way of phrasing her questions and thoughts abstractly. Her distinctive singsong tone tells you what she has in mind, often without her saying it explicitly. And before she asked, she knew precisely what we needed, and she made her thoughts known in a way that was not offensive, demanding, or threatening.

After the October summit meeting, she cornered me and asked, "Would a group of experts who could review and make recommendations to the OCME and New York State Police be valuable?" It was the word *valuable* that set her apart. The first time she said it, I had to ask myself, "What would be valuable?" Was I stupid? Of course, it would be valuable.

While running the risk of putting words in her mouth, I believe she was saying this: "The World Trade Center attacks were an important, historical event rivaling the attack on Pearl Harbor. Maybe you should have a group of respected scientists who can point you in the proper direction so that you do not do something stupid and embarrass yourselves or your agencies, while doing the right thing for your country. After all, history will judge what you do." In short, "Don't make an ass of yourself."

I heard her loud and clear. So did Mark. It was an admission, too, because my inclination is usually testosterone directed: "I can do this myself." Male hubris in action.

Then she asked, "What do you need?" She had approached the topic the first few times we met after 9/11, but this was the first time I was listening. My immediate concerns centered on software, and I said, "A group of experts who can help evaluate or find appropriate software would be extremely valuable."

Lisa immediately recognized my chaotic situation and knew the resources I needed. I can still remember her standing in the conference room in the OCME DNA laboratory. She looked directly at me, a twinkle in her eye, and said, for the second time, "If I can find the funding, I might be able to help." She smiled slightly and added, "No promises."

"I understand," I said, believing the money was on its way. Her words were music to my ears. As far as I was concerned, we had the funding for a panel of experts.

On October 10, the OCME and the New York State Police officially and jointly requested that the National Institute of Justice assemble a panel of experts to review, discuss, and advise us on the available kinship testing systems for associating the World Trade Center victims with their families. On October 18, 2001, we had the first Kinship and Data Analysis Panel, or KADAP, meeting at the Forensic Investigation Center in Albany. From that moment, this group assumed a central role in the World Trade Center DNA effort but received little or no recognition from politicians or the media and was relatively unknown outside the inner circle of the OCME, the New York State Police, and forensic industry and government Kinship and Data Analysis Panel members.

Lisa and I first met in the late 1980s. We were scientists working for competing private DNA companies; I was with Lifecodes Corporation and Lisa was with Cellmark Diagnostics. She represented a second wave of scientists on the DNA lecture circuit offering DNA services to the police and district attorneys around the country. We were the first to introduce DNA typing to the nation's criminal justice system.

A population geneticist by training, Lisa left Cellmark to take a position at the National Institute of Standards and Technology before joining the National Institute of Justice. Though I did not know her well when we met at the OCME in September 2001, I certainly respected her as a scientist. What I was rapidly learning was her proclivity for working through the governmental maze. She had an amazing understanding of the inner workings of, and had a penchant for accomplishing nearly impossible tasks within, the morass we call the federal government.

After receiving Mark's and my approval for forming a World Trade Center scientific working group, which she required, she approached her boss, Dr. David Boyd, and his boss, Sarah Hart. Sarah agreed to the idea and funneled funds previously allocated to other projects to the KADAP. This was a monumental decision by an in-touch and sensitive government official in ensuring the success of the World Trade Center DNA effort. It was also to the credit of the National Institute of Justice that it happened.

11 THE KINSHIP PANEL

October 31, 2001

Missing Identified: 193

DNA Identifications: 10

Remains Received: 8,655

Personal Effects at New York State Police: 3,354

We held the first Kinship and Data Analysis Panel meeting at the Forensic Investigation Center at the New York State Police in Albany, October 18 to 20, 2001. For that first meeting, Lisa had gathered a group of thirty-four scientists with expertise in human genetics, population genetics, statistics, high-volume throughput, parentage testing, kinship testing, mitochondrial genetics, DNA-based identification in mass disasters, forensics, information management, and legal and government affairs. These ingredients guaranteed a lively discussion. Lisa appointed National Institute of Justice contractor Dr. Amanda (Mandy) Sozer as facilitator, a role that suited Mandy's personality perfectly.

Dark haired and sporting a broad, sincere smile, Mandy is a mother of two children. She and I had met once before September 11 when she worked for the Fairfax Identity Laboratory, a high-throughput parentage and forensic testing laboratory. She and a colleague came to New York because they were interested in bidding on the New York City Police Department rape kit backlog project.

As I got to know her, I sometimes thought of Mandy as a benevolent pit bull. She's intense, focused, and determined. Additionally, she's intelligent, qualified, and delightful. With a background in molecular genetics, she has experience in forensic DNA testing, specifically STR testing. She also owns an independent DNA consulting business. She was a terrific choice to manage the diverse group of scientists that formed the Kinship and Data Analysis Panel. Keeping thirty-plus independent-minded and often opinionated scientists on track was not easy.

The scientists Lisa assembled represented universities, government, and private industry, including the NIH (the Human Genome Research Institute), National Center for Biological Informatics, Carleton University in Canada, the FBI, Yale University, Indiana University School of Medicine, University of North Texas, the National Institute of Justice, Myriad Genetic Laboratories, Harvard University, the Department of Defense DNA Registry (Armed Forces DNA Identification Laboratory), Gene Codes Forensics Corporation, OCME, New York State Police, New York City Police Department, and scientists working in the private sector.

I knew several of the panel members. The others I knew by reputation but had not met. I knew what I needed, but I feared that such a large group would get bogged down in philosophical and theoretical minutiae instead of concentrating on my needs. My immediate concern was getting to the point: I had to make DNA identifications. So far, I had none.

I still harbored personal doubts about my ability to manage the World Trade Center DNA effort, but at that moment I was more concerned with whether this group would consider me worthy. Their knowledge and experience base was astounding. I was humbled by it, yet honored to have them available. The university and government members of the Kinship and Data Analysis Panel were volunteers. No one paid them for their time, which was valuable, or for their expertise, which was priceless.

Shortly before this first KADAP conference, sometime in the third week of September, I was seeing problems in the STR typing of the DMs. I had no way of knowing what the final tabulation would be, but only about half of the samples were giving usable STR results because of the extreme damage done to the remains in the building collapses and subsequent fire. Eventually, the number of DMs giving borderline STR results would exceed 60 percent.

Lisa opened the meeting, made introductions, offered an overview of why we were there, and then turned the meeting over to Mandy. I was the first speaker. I confess I was as nervous as I have been in my entire life. Imagine being nervous and then nervous on top of that. That was me. I stood and faced the group. When I felt their eyes fix on me and saw their expectant faces, I felt inadequate and conspicuous. Everything I had planned to say suddenly evaporated in a weird brain sweep. I swallowed hard, then somehow managed to begin. In my opening remarks, I thanked everyone for coming. I certainly said more because I spoke for more than two seconds. I distinctly remember ending with "I need your help."

Actually, I remember presenting an overview of the World Trade Center DNA work, the current processes employed at the OCME with respect to human remains handling, and the problems we were having with computer networks and communication. I emphasized my concerns about obtaining appropriate matching and kinship software and also mentioned the poor STR results we were seeing from DMs.

Even at that early stage, I was thinking about alternative technologies, techniques that I thought might help later. The business of badly degraded DMs and the spotty STR test results we were seeing preyed on me throughout the two-day conference.

Lisa convened the KADAP to help us to evaluate available DNA-matching and kinship software. Howard and I had already decided to use the World Trade Center CODIS network to store STR data and to use its algorithms to make direct matches. We understood its limitations, but with no other options, it was the only way. It gave us a limited capability to make direct matches. We still could not perform kinship analysis, making it impossible for us to use DNA profiles obtained from family samples for identi-fications.

As I mentioned previously, CODIS was not designed for mass-fatality identifications, but we could use it to get started. Still, at the first KADAP meeting, I had this deep-seated wish that someone on the panel would stand up and say, "Hey, Bob, I just finished writing a terrific software package that does exactly what you want. I'll send it to you next week."

In truth, I had not expected anything so dramatic. In fact, I was surprised at myself for even fantasizing it might happen. Then I shocked myself at how depressed I was when it did not happen. Never underestimate the frailties of the human mind.

That first meeting defined the KADAP's role, as Mandy's official "goals" turned out to be much more aggressive than simply evaluating identification software. She had six goals that embraced current and future needs, including software. She had added mitochondrial DNA to the agenda, because I mentioned that mtDNA was important, sec-ond only to software. I had not mentioned, however, that mtDNA was a long way off in my planning. In the end, it was good to have mtDNA on the agenda. As it turned out, mitochondrial DNA, espe-cially how I was planning to use it for the World Trade Center work, would rack the panel's intellect for an entire year.

Mandy's first KADAP agenda fully consumed both days. As for software solutions for making identifications, Dr. Charles Brenner, Dr. Benoit Leclair, Dr. Tom Parsons (Armed Forces DNA Identifica-tion Lab), and Dr. Ed Huffine (International Commission on Missing Persons, formerly of the Armed Forces DNA Identification Lab) pre-sented the essence of the human-identification software packages they were using or had used in mass disasters.

Ed came from Bosnia to share the software he had developed for identifying the dead found in mass graves there. The morning before the conference, the BBC interviewed Ed, two of his Bosnian col-leagues, and me in a hotel room at the Dumont Plaza (now the Affinia Dumont) on 34th Street in Manhattan. The interview had to be in the hotel room because, for security reasons, the OCME refused to allow reporters into the building or even near the 30th Street morgue. There was also the concern that photos or video of the remains would end up on television or in a newspaper.

I was a little unhappy with the interview. As it was edited and aired on the BBC, it seemed like I was interested in acquiring the International Committee for Missing Persons software. As it turned out, I was not. When Ed demonstrated how the software worked to the Kinship and Data Analysis Panel, I realized it was not ready for what I needed. It had not been designed to address the problems I was anticipating from the World Trade Center samples, though it did track samples and do direct matching. It would have to be adapted to the specific needs of the World Trade Center work. I was already having logistical problems, so the idea of designing software from both sides of the Atlantic Ocean was not appealing.

Next, Charles Brenner discussed DNAView. He also gave an interesting theoretical account of how he envisioned screening mass disasters for kinship matches, which, typically, flew against the conventional wisdom espoused by the FBI. I was intrigued by his approach, and knowing Charles as I did, I was pleased and not at all surprised by his unorthodox approach. However, like the Bosnia software, DNAView was not ready. There was a difference, though. Charles was already under contract to the OCME, and we could expand that contract to include DNAView upgrades. Knowing I had Charles in the fold made me feel a lot better.

Benoit Leclair's program was an Excel spreadsheet that he used for the Swissair crash when he was with the Royal Canadian Mounted Police Laboratory. His approach was a pairwise comparison, which was similar to the one the FBI proposed for WTC CODIS. Our experience from a small sampling of World Trade Center data showed that working with CODIS to make kinship matches was not feasible. While Benoit's program appeared to have the mountain of data under control, his first sampling of World Trade Center data was housed in boxes and contained more than 1,200 pages. Going through the data was overwhelming, but we had already decided to use Benoit's program in conjunction with DNAView.

Dr. Tom Parsons presented LISA (Laboratory Information Systems Application), the Armed Forces DNA Identification Lab's software used for identifying the Pennsylvania and Pentagon September 11 victims. The program looked robust; however, it too was unable to handle the multiple comparisons needed for the World Trade Center work. What it did, it did well, but I was not sure how we would get the program updated to meet our needs. At the time, there did not appear to be a simple mechanism to accomplish this.

Then Tom announced that he'd already identified more than one hundred people who had died at the Pentagon and at Shanksville, Pennsylvania. Their task was not really complex, but his announcement shocked me, and my mood soured instantly. I had thousands to identify, but as we sat there, I had yet to identify a single victim using DNA. It was disheartening and frustrating.

After the software overviews I found myself at exactly the same place I had been after the summit meeting weeks earlier. I thought maybe something might have happened between that meeting and the first KADAP conference, that someone had found a workable solution.

Also, I was hearing two approaches to the kinship problem, and I was torn between them. Seeing benefit from both, I had already made up my mind to use both DNAView and Benoit's program, which he later called MDKAP (Mass Disaster Kinship Analysis Program). My plan was to have one program back up the other.

Equally problematic, however, was the critical issue of obtaining both programs. I felt fairly certain I could get DNAView, but I was not confident of MDKAP because of problems I had heard—rumors only—with the Royal Canadian Mounted Police.

Then the Kinship and Data Analysis Panel moved on to mtDNA.

What happened completely surprised me. An intense discussion developed over the use of mitochondrial DNA and the company I had chosen to perform the work. I was shocked when the NIH members of the panel excused themselves and left the room. I was peripherally aware of the conflict between the public and private efforts to sequence the human genome, but I had not realized how deep-rooted those feelings were.

Not only that, but the topic of mitochondrial DNA evoked an as yet unspoken hostility with respect to mtDNA and how I planned to use it. While the open debate centered on the appropriate use of mtDNA sequencing, I sensed the discussion had much deeper overtones. Thinking back on my September 28 meeting with Howard Cash and his staff, I remembered sensing that he was not fond of Celera.

Unknowingly, by bringing Celera into my World Trade Center fold to sequence mitochondrial DNA, I had opened a parcel of potential problems. I also quickly learned that Celera was not my only mtDNA issue. Chuck Hirsch wanted us to mitotype *all* the disaster and kinship samples. Tom Parsons, a recognized expert in employing mtDNA sequencing in mass-fatality incidents and someone who probably had more experience than anyone at the meeting in analyzing mitochondrial DNA in compromised tissue and bone, argued persuasively against this approach. He firmly believed we would create more problems than we would solve. Mitochondrial DNA has inherent scientific issues that must be resolved, and Tom argued that because of this, we ran the risk of developing conflicting identification data.

Everyone in the room understood that mitotypes alone would not be sufficient to make individual identifications, but Tom's other concerns were sticky issues, topics that consumed subsequent Kinship and Data Analysis Panel meetings and a mitochondrial DNA subpanel for months.

As the second morning wore on, I worried that many of my concerns would remain unanswered. Mandy sensed this, and after lunch, she pulled me aside and said, "What else do you want the panel to consider?" At future Kinship and Data Analysis Panel meetings, Mandy and sometimes Lisa always asked me the same question.

"I need statistical cutoffs for direct and kinship matches," I said.

It was no secret that the first phase of testing would employ STRs as the dominant DNA testing technology. However, with CODIS the FBI had never distributed guidelines for making matches, except to infer that a match of the accepted thirteen loci was equivalent to identifying an unknown person. Each profile had a statistical "rarity," or likelihood ratio that could be calculated from population frequencies. The thirteen-locus matching guideline, although unwritten, worked for the criminal justice system. For the World Trade Center work, matching DMs at thirteen loci would be the easy part. Unfortunately, most of the DMs were not yielding 13 loci, many not even close and many none at all.

That was my dilemma.

I was in uncharted territory. We needed a statistical floor, a minimum threshold, for making identifications. No forensic DNA laboratory in the United States had established guidelines for making identifications using fewer than thirteen loci. Many questions were swarming inside my head. How many loci did I need? Ten? Six?

I left the first Kinship and Data Analysis Panel with several recommendations. There was an overview statement:

> The Panel recognizes the unprecedented complexity of identifying the victims from the World Trade Center attacks. They further recognize the expertise of the OCME, the New York City Police Department, and the New York State Police. The Panel stresses that, given the evolving nature of the task of identifying victims, these initial recommendations may be modified by OCME, New York City Police Department, or New York State Police, as deemed necessary and appropriate to the circumstances. The Panel remains available to the OCME, New York City Police Department, and New York State Police for consultation upon request.
>
> After review of the available systems, the Panel agreed that no single software program currently exists that meets

all of the analytical needs for resolution of the identity of World Trade Center victims.

I never understood why the panel included the New York City Police Department in the recommendation statement because the NYPD had nothing to do with the World Trade Center DNA work and did not have the expertise to change or modify any of the panel's recommendations. I guessed it was politics. As expected, the panel recognized that the prevailing forensic standard, a thirteen-loci match of the CODIS loci, would be sufficient to report an identification. A recommendation to use CODIS in the short term to make direct matches was what Howard Baum and I had already decided on and had begun using.

The panel, however, recommended using a likelihood ratio (a statistical match standard) of 1×10^{10} (one in 10 billion). This value came from Charles Brenner, who responded to me. When asked what error rate we would tolerate, I said, "None." Charles said that, if we were 99 percent certain of a match, we needed a 1-in-10 billion matching frequency to guarantee no errors at this level of certainty. This was important. For the first time, STRs had a statistical basis for identifying someone with less than the full CODIS thirteen-loci profile. It was a mechanism for us to use partially degraded DMs. Practically, the panel's recommendation meant that a ten-locus profile would normally suffice to reach this level of certainty. This alleviated my fears that at some future date I would be hauled into court to explain my reasoning. Not that it could not happen. It certainly could, but I would have the support of the panel. I would not be alone.

For kinship identifications, the panel suggested using DNAView at a minimum probability of relationship of 99.9 percent. The panel set what geneticists call the prior probability at 1 in 5,000 (to reflect then current estimates of the World Trade Center missing population size). I could change the prior probability in case-by-case situations or if the estimated number of missing changed. Thankfully, over time, the number would fall. This was also a critical recommendation because I could theoretically begin making identifications using the kinship swabs taken from the relatives of the missing person.

Also, I had anticipated the panel's thoughts on mtDNA. It recommended using the existing mass-fatality paradigm: sequencing victim samples only as a last resort and only after reanalysis and/or the use of additional forensically validated STRs. The panel suggested using Y chromosomes or other nuclear markers as a first choice. In this recommendation, the Kinship and Data Analysis Panel was saying, in essence, that it did not agree with the approach to test all of the World Trade Center samples for mtDNA.

The panel went further, however, saying mtDNA typing should be done on all appropriate maternal lineage samples using a suitable validated system. In a backhanded way, I believe the KADAP was telling me that Celera had not been a wise choice because, at the time of the meeting, the company did not yet have a forensically validated mtDNA procedure.

Another KADAP recommendation demonstrated the panel's awareness of what might lie in the future. We had discussed degraded DNA and the possible use of new technology, a topic that had been on my mind during the conference. The recommendation centered on new, untried methods that might prove useful. The panel said that if currently available forensically validated systems are not sufficient to resolve identity, then research-grade systems should be explored on a case-by-case basis.

This was a critical concession. The panel recognized that the World Trade Center work, though still an ongoing forensic and criminal investigation, might not neatly fall under the federal guidelines for routine criminal forensic DNA testing.

Howard Baum and I realized that mtDNA and STRs alone might not suffice to make all the identifications. Though I did not know what these new technologies might be, I needed this respected group to agree that something else might be needed. Of the nine recommendations, this was the second most important.

On October 20, I left the first KADAP conference feeling much more secure about my chances to succeed. I had a lot yet to do, but my DNA program was falling into place. We would use CODIS for direct matches. Howard Cash's company had accepted the critical role of writing software to replace CODIS and to incorporate mtDNA sequence data into it. I had DNAView, but I still needed a robust kinship software program. When it came—if it came—the panel had provided me with the statistical foundation to make those identifications, too.

The most disturbing outcome of the KADAP centered on the use of mtDNA. The panel was steadfastly against high-volume mtDNA sequencing. Celera's forte was high-volume DNA sequencing, although not specifically mtDNA sequencing. However, it was this high-volume capability that led me to choose the company. I was beginning to have second thoughts about the choice. I had placed myself at odds with a significantly important group of the scientific community.

There was also a media issue I had to deal with, because Celera had leaked to the print media that it would have a significant role in the World Trade Center work. This placed me in an awkward situation. I had to field questions from persistent reporters clamoring for nuggets to print. Celera was one such nugget, and I carefully avoided the Kinship and Data Analysis Panel controversy with respect to mitochondrial DNA. It was tempting, though, if only to shut up Celera's publicity-hungry executives. Controversy aside, if not Celera, then who? For my money, the company was the only game in town.

The Kinship and Data Analysis Panel met every other month, nine times in all, the last occurring in June 2005 after a time delay since September 2003, when the National Institute of Justice money dried up. I believe every major mass-fatality event would benefit from a group of scientists like this. For the World Trade Center DNA effort, which had such a complex technological basis, the panel proved invaluable.

On the afternoon of the second day of the KADAP, something inspiring happened. After lunch, Mandy had just brought the group to order when Karen Dooling came beaming into the conference room and ran up to me. I could not imagine what she wanted. She leaned over and whispered, "We have our first real match!"

I couldn't believe it. We had our first identification! I had to fight back the tears.

She and I left the conference room and hustled downstairs to the New York State Police CODIS room and then waited for Peter Wistort, the State Police CODIS manager, to analyze the data. Though he had a ton of additional work to do before officially releasing the identification to Karen, it was a start. We were rolling. It was a very good feeling.

I called Chuck Hirsch.

12 THE "BIG MINI"

The DNA we were getting from the tissue and bones recovered from the World Trade Center site was getting progressively worse. The DNA was degrading rapidly, a stark truth I had been aware of since the latter part of September 2001. The reality was that once DNA degrades completely, it is gone, irretrievable. I needed a way to coerce these badly compromised tissues and bones to give up their genetic secrets. A more sobering thought prevailed: would we ever know who these DMs came from? I had to do something.

In looking at the DNA data, I had reason to hope. The DNA in some of these tissues and bones was grudgingly yielding partial STR results, although insufficient to make identifications, to be sure, and insufficient to meet the Kinship and Data Analysis Panel statistical barrier. However, the mere presence of partial STR results offered the slimmest hope that all was not lost. The fact that DNA, which is an extremely long molecule, degrades progressively into smaller and smaller fragments was the clue.

My next step actually had its roots back in July 2000. My laboratory had a monthly journal club where one of my scientists presented the findings of a scientific publication. In July 2000, I presented an alternative method of analysis, different from what we were doing in our laboratory: mass spectrometry for the analysis of STRs. It was another way to obtain STR results.

Mass spectrometry is traditionally used to analyze the molecular structure of small molecules, like drugs or the products of metabolism. It has historically had a relatively poor track record with larger molecules, like proteins and nucleic acids, such as DNA and RNA. However, the technique was showing promise for nucleic acids.

While looking for a topic for the journal club back then, I contacted Dr. John Butler, then a scientist working at Gene-Trace Systems, Inc. Always accommodating, he had sent me mass-spectrometry data on DNA and other publication information that I used.

Dr. John Butler's magic lies in his genius. He had figured out how to use mass spectrometry to analyze STRs. Unlike many contemporary scientists, especially those in industry, John is all about science for the public. He believes in solving problems to get an answer, not for financial reward or to obtain a patent to augment a corporate bottom line. At GeneTrace, John had designed a system for STRs that I thought could be used to analyze degraded DNA better than those obtained from commercially available STR-typing kits.

Most forensic STR typing in the United States utilizes commercially available forensic DNA typing kits because they produce a reliable and quick DNA result without having to manufacture the critical ingredients, the reagents.

The process of obtaining an STR test involves obtaining test results at specific regions of the DNA, each of which is an independent STR. In order to accomplish this, it is necessary to utilize a technique called the polymerase chain reaction (PCR), where the specific regions of interest on the DNA are specifically targeted and then amplified (copied) millions of times. These copies are fragments of DNA called amplicons, the size of which is the issue of this discussion. The size of the DNA amplicons produced using the commercial kits varies from 100 to approximately 400 base pairs.

This meant that if the DNA fragment from a DM was smaller than 400 base pairs, the PCR reaction would yield either partial STR profiles or no profiles, depending on the extent of degradation. This is precisely what we were seeing.

Many of the tissue and bone DMs were yielding only amelogenin (approximately 100 base pairs), the sexing locus, or nothing. Another subset of World Trade Center samples was yielding minimal STR-typing information, upwards of approximately 200 base pairs. This meant I was losing loci to degradation, so I was looking for an

STR test that could examine the thirteen CODIS loci but do it on amplicons of approximately 100 base pairs.

An example from the early World Trade Center work involved a DM, a piece of tissue recovered from the WTC site that had been exposed to such heat that it came into the lab charred and dried. This turned out to be a particularly important DM because it supposedly came from a firefighter whose wife was the secretary of an important public official. Late one afternoon, the official came to the OCME wanting the identification made as quickly as possible. He returned at 2:00 A.M. to monitor our progress. It was a pressured situation. On first glance, we doubted there was usable DNA in the tissue. We had to analyze the sample, so Pat Buffolino stayed in the lab all night. After multiple attempts, the tissue reluctantly gave up only six loci. This happened before the first Kinship and Data Analysis Panel meeting, so we did not have a defined statistical cutoff. The statistical rarity of the six loci obtained was 1 in 110,000, which was not good enough to make the identification. Fortunately for the family, we had personal information that had been recovered with the remains which, coupled with the DNA, was sufficient to make the ID.

For DMs like this, where there were missing loci, however, adding back loci would be critical to returning a high percentage of the remains where other personal information was unavailable. In the above instance, the missing eight (thirteen CODIS loci plus one sexing locus, amelogenin) loci were in the 200-to-400 base pair range. I was looking for a way to add these loci back, "fill in the blanks," so to speak. If I could add back even four of the eight missing loci—since generally ten were sufficient to meet the KADAP's statistical barrier—we would have had sufficient genetic information for DNA alone to have made the ID.

Even before the first KADAP meeting, I was struggling for a way to analyze these compromised samples. I remembered John's work at GeneTrace but knew he was no longer working there. I wondered whether his concept was worth a try. I decided to get another opinion. At the October 2001 KADAP, I asked Lisa Forman what she thought. She said it was worth a try. She knew that John was working at the National Institute of Science and Technology and sent me his contact information. I'm not sure of the exact date I called, but John sent me an e-mail on November 5 indicating that he had already spoken to Lisa. I was elated. Apparently, when he joined the National Institute of Science and Technology, he revived his GeneTrace work and adapted it to the current forensic instrumental platform, the same one we were using for the World Trade Center work. This was great news.

I had been on an emotional roller coaster for weeks, so his next statement was sobering and, admittedly, a bit demoralizing. He had stopped working with the system, which he called "miniplexes" (named for the smaller—mini—amplicons that could be run multiply in the same reaction vessel). He had to pursue more pressing needs. My heart fell. I wondered whether that meant the idea was not feasible or that the National Institute of Science and Technology would not allow him to pursue it.

As I listened, my spirits rose again. He believed the concept would work with decomposing tissues. When he offered to expedite this work and prioritize it, my heart soared. He expected it would take six to eight weeks to finish the validation.

John's work was further along than I had originally thought. He had already adapted the thirteen CODIS STRS to the new format, which was exactly what I needed. Also, he had redesigned the test by reworking the thirteen into logical groups of three to four loci each, giving him six groups, or miniplexes. One particularly relevant miniplex had six loci, the same ones routinely missing in degraded DNA. John called this "the Big Mini."

I wanted the Big Mini.

On January 3, 2002, Howard Baum sent me an e-mail after speaking with John. He had finished the Big Mini design and was working on validating the test. I was thrilled.

• • •

Later in that January, John, Howard Baum, and I gave presentations at the FBI in Quantico, Virginia, at the annual Scientific Working Group for DNA Methods meeting. A group of forensic biologists sponsored by the FBI to formulate policy with respect to forensic DNA testing, they were originally called the Technical Working Group for DNA Analysis Methods. It was formed in the early days of forensic DNA testing in the United States to study DNA methods and suggest quality guidelines. It was the first time my forensic colleagues would learn anything about our World Trade Center DNA work. Howard spoke first and described our work in identifying the victims of American Airlines Flight 587, which had gone down in the Rockaways in Queens, New York, exactly two months and a day after September 11.

Then it was my turn.

I walked to the lectern, looked over the group, and then promptly lost every thought I ever had. This was becoming a disturbing trend. Naturally, I panicked. But having gone down this path before, I knew what to do. I took a deep breath.

No one in the room knew what had been happening in New York with respect to our work except for what they had seen and read in the media. I knew they would be curious. Before the meeting, several people had mentioned having heard this or that about it; no one had been close. These were my friends, my peers, and my colleagues, many of whom could be outspoken and critical, so I was apprehensive. That's their job and why they were there. Also, many of them are quite dogmatic. They believe forensic DNA should be done in a certain way.

They would soon learn we had stepped out of the so-called forensic DNA box with plans to move out further. I was expecting questions like, "Why are you doing it like that?" or, "Why not try this?" or "Did you think of this?"

I gave my presentation. When I finished, I looked out over the group and steeled myself for the onslaught. There was dead silence. If I remember correctly, no one asked a question. These curious-minded people always ask questions. Always! Were they appalled? Were they in awe? I returned to my seat, stunned.

Next it was John Butler's turn to talk. I had not yet seen his final validation on the Big Mini. This was my moment of truth. It was also a moment of truth for the World Trade Center families. I had no idea what he would say. The only inkling I had was what he said during our conversation in November. Maybe he had proven the miniplex concept would not work, although I believed he would have called if there were major problems. Still, I was praying. I had placed my personal reputation on the miniplex concept, even knowing that no one had tried it on true-grit forensic samples. The World Trade Center DMs represented the ultimate in forensic testing.

John approached the lectern. I listened carefully as he spoke. He showed that the size range of analyzable DNA using miniplexes ranged from 89 to 218 base pairs. When he finished, I was feeling really, really good. Although he had not yet worked with World Trade Center samples, I thought his system should work. Especially with those DMs that were partially degraded. I was impressed with the Big Mini.

13 AN ALTERNATIVE ARRIVES ON THE SCENE

Sometime in the fall of 2001, after I had spoken with John Butler in November, I couldn't shake the feeling that I might need more than the Big Mini. I believed John Butler's concept of miniplexes certainly offered a reasonable approach to solving the problem of degraded DNA, but I wasn't convinced it was the only answer. I was particularly concerned about those DMs whose average fragment size was in the 100–base pair range.

John's presentation in January 2002 had turned me on to the potential of the miniplexes, which I believed offered a reasonable chance to resurrect many DMs that had already given a partial DNA profile. However, in October and November 2001, before John had finished his validation, I could not predict how well the miniplexes would work, so I was looking for something else, a second iron in the fire. I felt like I was always looking for a second iron in the fire.

After the first Kinship and Data Analysis Panel meeting in October, I started thinking seriously about SNPs. They were the smallest variation on DNA and I wondered whether they might offer a viable alternative to STR typing for degraded DMs.

The smallest structural element on the DNA ladder is the rung, or base pair. An SNP (single nucleotide polymorphism) is a variation at a specific base pair. As a result, an SNP represents a difference among people at the most basic and smallest level of the DNA molecule: the individual building unit, the base pair, the rung of the ladder.

For years before September 11, I had been reading and hearing about something called the SNP Consortium, which was a group of scientists and organizations in the pharmaceutical industry that was looking at SNPs for drug-sensitivity studies. The prevailing thought was that a person's sensitivity to drugs could be ascertained genetically and demonstrated empirically. Since there are literally thousands of SNPs, they were a logical choice for these investigations.

Once a new technique surfaces, everyone wants a shot at it. I call it the herd effect because if you failed to publish on the new and sexiest scientific fad, you were quickly outdated. Forensic scientists are no different. The European forensic community, especially, had been considering using SNPs for human identification and casework applications as either an alternative or an add-on to STRs.

Before September 11, conversations about forensic applications of SNPs were mostly theoretical. No public forensic DNA laboratory in the United States was using them or even considering incorporating them into casework. Since most public forensic laboratories in the States tend to follow the FBI's lead, there was little chance SNPs would be used extensively anytime soon. There were good reasons for this. The SNP data is completely different from STR data. Also, there would have to be extensive validation of the technology in forensic situations before SNPs could be used in casework.

There were questions to be answered. Which SNPs would be forensically appropriate, or how many would be the equivalent of a thirteen-locus STR match? There were literally thousands of SNPs from which to choose. There were technical problems such as interpreting mixtures. Sorting these out would not be trivial.

From what I could see, the largest hurdle was CODIS. No American forensic DNA laboratory would spend the time or the expense bringing SNPs online unless the data could be uploaded to CODIS. Our entire American DNA network was STR based, so forensic DNA labs were pretty much locked into them. Also, CODIS is an

FBI tool, which meant the agency would be unlikely to switch completely over to SNPs. Still, SNPs appealed to me.

I had the formidable task of working with DMs that had been chopped into extremely small pieces because of the extensive decomposition of the World Trade Center remains. If I could find someone who could design an SNP test so that the largest fragment of DNA required to get a result was less than 100 base pairs, I might have a chance of analyzing the more extensively degraded DNA when STRs, especially miniplexes—if they worked at all—failed, which was inevitable when the average size of the DNA became too small.

From the World Trade Center data I was receiving from Bode, Myriad, and our in-house work, a large percentage of the World Trade Center samples were giving little or no STR data.

I had a fleeting thought that using SNPs might have more merit than mtDNA. However, Celera was already on board, so I could not back out. As it would happen, I got lucky. Had I known what the future held, I might have had second thoughts. In a state of ignorant bliss, once again I asked Lisa Forman for help. Once again, she pointed me in the right direction. In her role at the National Institute of Justice, Lisa was plugged into emerging DNA technologies. I figured she could help find a laboratory or company that controlled—had patented—the largest number of SNPs.

SNPs turned out to be a controversial idea, which I learned as soon as I mentioned the project to the KADAP. Lisa was supportive and thought the idea had merit. Thank God! I needed someone outside the OCME family with credibility who shared my vision. And once again she pointed me in the right direction.

My strategy to analyze degraded DNA, at least for the foreseeable future, ended when I included SNPs in my analytical equation. I had mtDNA, John Butler's Big Mini, and now SNPs. These were conceptually three different approaches to the problem. While I expected the Big Mini would give good results on a certain, unknowable percentage of the degraded DMs, our early data suggested as many as 28 percent of the samples might not. I wanted a legitimate shot at putting names to the DMs having fewer than 100 base pairs remaining. I reasoned that the DNA in these was not completely destroyed. I was banking that SNPs gave me that chance.

Lisa suggested I call Cellmark Diagnostics, now Orchid Cellmark. Orchid owned (patented) hundreds of SNPs. I spoke to Mark Stolorow, executive director, who mentioned that his former competitor, GeneScreen in Dallas—now a part of the Orchid Cellmark family of laboratories—had developed an SNP paternity test. I was elated. Not only did it appear that I might have access to a test that might be almost ready to go, but it was being developed by a laboratory I knew well.

Orchid Cellmark in Dallas—then GeneScreen—and Cellmark in Germantown, Maryland, had contracts with the New York City Police Department to help process those seventeen thousand backlogged rape kits. I had a good working relationship with Dr. Bob Giles, the general manager of the Orchid Dallas laboratory. I also knew many on his scientific staff. When I spoke to him on November 13, I felt like I was in familiar territory.

Bob confirmed what Mark had said. His laboratory had developed an SNP paternity test. That was the good news. When I explained what I needed, I heard the bad news. The conversation turned out to be an emotional up and down, much like when I first spoke to John Butler about miniplexes.

First, my heart sank. Bob mentioned that the size of the amplicon fragments in the Orchid SNP paternity test were mostly larger than 100 base pairs. The SNP paternity test, in its current format, would not be useful for analyzing DMs.

"Can you redesign the test so that the size of the amplicons is less than one hundred base pairs?" I asked.

There was silence. "I think we can, but I'll have to run it by Princeton," he said, referring to Orchid's headquarters in Princeton, New Jersey.

I had no doubt it could be done. It was really a matter of what the company wanted to do. I remember thinking that Orchid did not have a choice. If they wanted their name associated with the World Trade Center project, they would find a way to do what I wanted. In fall 2001, many companies were craving to be associated with the World Trade Center effort. Orchid was suffering financial losses, as I later learned from a newspaper article, so they probably felt that working on the World Trade Center project would enhance their image. On November 12, I had no idea that their financial position was shaky. Had I known, I might have asked Lisa for another SNP source.

During our conversation, I asked Bob to choose an SNP panel that did not link with the CODIS STRs or to each other. This would be critical if we were going to use SNPs for kinship analysis, which I knew we would have to do eventually. He agreed, saying he would ask Princeton to come up with a usable panel of SNPs.

I thought I had found another test with the potential of obtaining genomic DNA (as opposed to mitochondrial DNA) from badly degraded DMs. The bad news was that the test had to be completely redesigned and then validated, which would take time. I didn't know how much. Again, if I had, I might have changed my mind about pursuing the test. Ignorance proved to be bliss.

That's when I went into Mecki's office and found out what Howard thought of the idea.

To my dismay, not everyone was enthusiastic about the idea. I bounced it off of Howard Baum, as I usually did. Howard was a perfect foil because we often did not see eye to eye. I have always valued his thoughts because they often tempered my enthusiasm. He and I were in Mecki's office when I brought up the subject of SNPs. I explained what I was thinking. The first words out of Howard's mouth took me completely by surprise: "It won't work."

Mecki held her counsel. At first, I was stunned. Then I was angry. Howard's negative attitude toward the idea really galled me, and I lost it. "Why are you always so negative?" I challenged.

He stammered for an instant, then said, "It can't do mixtures.

There are too many mixtures"—this was a reference to commingling and a perception, at the time, of contamination—"in the Trade Center samples."

Howard had and may still harbor the opinion that most of the World Trade Center DMs were mixtures. Speculating that this was true, given how the buildings fell and how people died together, might be reasonable. However, I had reviewed thousands of STR profiles and had not seen enough mixtures to suggest this was a problem. Not enough, anyway, to dampen my enthusiasm for SNPs. I guessed perhaps as many as 10 percent of the DMs were STR mixtures. Even if the number were larger, I did not believe this was sufficient reason to forgo doing SNPs.

Howard was not going to back me, at least privately. He thought the miniplexes had been a good idea. When push came to shove, Howard did back me publicly, setting aside his personal skepticism. I certainly had no crystal ball with respect to SNPs, but I thought it was worth a try. Howard actually agreed.

14 THEIR LIVES MATTERED

November 30, 2001

Missing Identified: 265

DNA Identifications: 55

Remains Received: 10,055

Personal Effects at New York State Police: 3,429

The logline beside James Marcel Cartier's photo in the book *Portraits 2001*, which collected the obituaries of WTC victims, reads, "The More Work, the Better." James was a young man whose infective personality highlighted his zest for life. He was a special person who touched the lives of those around him."

Sadly, I never met James Cartier. But I do know him. I know the kind of man he was because I know his family. At twenty-six, he was an apprentice electrician who had been assigned to the World Trade Center just two weeks before the attacks

I met James's father, Patrick Cartier, on December 10, 2001, on the telephone. Although I didn't know it at the time, the call would change my life.

Katie Sullivan is a wonderfully compassionate woman who was Shiya Ribowsky's right-hand person. She worked "in the conference room" with the other medicolegal investigators, where all of the World Trade Center data converged. Katie came to New York from Oregon to help out with the World Trade Center work as a DMORT volunteer. She planned to stay just two weeks. Over time, she became the World Trade Center supervisor for identifications, taking over for Shiya. Her trademark was the compassion she showed grieving families, which allowed her to forge tight and lasting bonds with them. She worked with the families day in and day out for more than three years. She made the difficult phone calls. The process took its toll, and she left the World Trade Center work at the end of April 2005 emotionally drained.

She called and asked if I would speak to an outraged family member who had lost his son. She continued, "Mr. Cartier has questions about DNA that I can't answer."

Katie gave me what scant information she had about James Cartier, which amounted only to New York City Police Department tracking numbers for his personal effects and the OCME data the family had provided to the NYPD when at a Family Assistance Center. There was nothing else. The remainder of the Cartier family data was in Albany with the NYSP. I did not have direct access to it.

Coincidentally, earlier that week I had met Patrick's daughter, Jennie Farrell, at a meeting of family members and World Trade Center funding groups at the Mayor's Office of Community Affairs. The meeting was at best contentious and, at times, explosive. The chasm between the members of the service (including the New York City Fire Department, the New York City Police Department, Emergency Services, and Port Authority Police) and civilian families had grown. By this time, the civilian families were frustrated by what they considered preferential treatment of members of service families, and they had gone to the media to force their case.

The civilian families wanted the same treatment for their loved ones as the members of service families received. Additionally, extreme anger born from grief was being directed at the Office of Emergency Management and the mayor. I had been reading about the problem in the tabloids and heard about it on TV news broadcasts. But seeing how these families perceived how they were being treated by the mayor and the press was an eye-opener. As I sat there with Chuck Hirsch, I feared their wrath would soon descend on us. The

OCME was not part of that fight, I hoped. Jennie Farrell, James Cartier's sister, had become the spokesperson for the group.

When I lifted the phone to call Patrick, I was nervous. At this point, I had not had the opportunity to speak with many families, perhaps eight or ten, and in each instance, they had been extremely polite and appreciative of our work. Chuck Hirsch and I had attended a couple of family meetings in Mayor Giuliani's office, where the mayor's presence seemed to shield us. Chuck has a calming influence on people. Unfortunately, I do not possess that talent.

I remember thinking that Chuck would not be with me when I called Patrick. Katie Sullivan had mentioned that he was threatening to go to the newspapers about a problem she was sure I could solve. Frankly, I was intimidated. I was still reeling from the meeting with Jennie and the other angry family members.

With trepidation I dialed Patrick's number. It rang only twice. A man answered. I swallowed hard. "I am Dr. Shaler with the Medical Examiner's Office. May I speak with Patrick Cartier?"

What followed was a conversation with a man in anguish, a man grieving for his lost son. He assaulted me with a barrage of information about his Korean War record and lost family samples, then ended with a threat to go to the newspapers if I did not answer his questions. I wanted to run and hide. I empathized with him. Patrick had every right to feel the way he did.

It turns out, Patrick had given an oral swab at Pier 94 as part of the NYPD collection of family kin samples. From a recent article he had read in the *New York Post*, he believed the OCME had lost his swab. The *Post* article said that the OCME was reaching out to families because a number of the samples did not have sufficient information to make identifications. The article did not mention we had lost the family samples. However, a grieving family might have reached that conclusion.

I held the phone to my ear. I had looked up everything I could find about James Cartier, and I thought I was ready. I was not. In the end, all Patrick Cartier wanted was some assurance that we had what we needed to find his son. It was a reasonable request. I did not have the answer to his question and felt that I had let him down. The information he wanted was supposed to be in Albany at the State Police lab, which is precisely what I explained to him.

I don't know whether he believed me, and I hoped he did not think I was stalling. To his credit, he gave me the benefit of the doubt. I promised I would call him with the information before the day ended.

I hung up the phone and took a deep breath. I prayed Peter Wistort was at work because he was my only contact at the State Police for the information. I dreaded the thought of having to call Patrick back to tell him he would have to wait another day.

I called Albany.

Peter was there, thank God. I told him what I wanted and then held while he looked up the information. After a couple of minutes, he gave me everything he had about James: his birth date; a P number, which was an NYPD family number; a T number, which was an NYPD family number given after a phone call; an NYPD DNA collection number; and a WDI number, which the State Police assigned to family samples they obtained.

"Do you have the father's swab?" I asked.

"Yes," Peter said. "It has a full DNA profile."

I shut my eyes. "That's great news. Thanks, Peter."

I had been looking in God's direction a lot in those days, so I must have looked skyward. We had Patrick's DNA, and it was a full STR profile. However, Peter had some disconcerting news, too. We had collected samples from only James's father, which meant we had only Patrick's DNA. The other members of his family had not donated. I do not know why, but I suspected it was because of faulty information given to the family when they came to the Family Assistance Center. The bottom line for Patrick, and me, was that, even if we had recovered James's remains and had obtained an STR profile from them, we could not have IDed him. When I lifted the phone to call Patrick back, I wondered how he would accept that.

I reached Patrick and explained the situation. There was silence on the other end of the phone. When he finally spoke, he was in complete control and apparently satisfied that he had been given a chance to speak to someone in charge, someone who had answers.

He thanked me. "What do I have to do?" he asked.

"I need DNA from James's mother, and it wouldn't hurt to have samples from his brothers and sisters," I said, knowing James had six siblings.

Though I did not know it at the time, my conversation with Patrick had initiated a change inside of me that would take months to mature. My mission to identify the missing was becoming an obsession. This was the second time I had experienced the absolute anguish of a family member who had lost a loved one.

The first time was at the Mayor's Office of Consumer Affairs, the meeting where I first met Patrick's daughter, Jennie. A distraught young man screamed at Richie Scherer, then the Director of the Office of Emergency Management (OEM) in the Giuliani administration, about the handling of bodies at the World Trade Center site and then stormed out of the room, accusing Richie of being a liar.

Nothing could have been further from the truth. Richie is one of the most compassionate and honest men I have had the honor of meeting. The city owes him a debt of gratitude for the work he did during September 11 and its aftermath.

However, at that meeting, the young man was only one of many family members, Jennie included, who were angry. Jennie had been the most visible, having been often quoted in the press and on network news. She and the other members of her family founded Give Your Voice, one of the most outspoken and influential of the family groups, dedicated to the rights of the civilians who lost their loved ones at the World Trade Center.

The families had legitimate questions about the rescue and recovery process. They wanted information, and they wanted to be included in the administration's information flow. What they were getting was misinformation from the print and broadcast media. They wanted the truth, no matter how difficult it was to bear.

That was the message I carried back to my laboratory. Truth. It became my credo in discussions I had with families. They were prepared to deal with it.

There had been innuendos and rumors about body collection: the recovery of remains from the World Trade Center site and the Staten Island Fresh Kills landfill, birds flying away with body pieces at the landfill, preferential treatment of uniformed service members over missing civilians, and a litany of sensitive topics. The truth was all the families wanted and believing they were not getting it was the root of their anger. Getting the runaround, if only perceived, fueled their mistrust.

This was also the first time I learned of the semantic issue surrounding the recovery of "intact" bodies. The press continually reported the recovery of intact bodies, while the remains coming to the OCME were anything but intact. This issue festered for months.

As Chuck and I were leaving the meeting, I mentioned Jennie. I said, "I'm glad I'm not married to her." He only smiled. Jennie would become a dear and valued friend. When I later told her husband, Dan, the story, he laughed.

While I was able to get James Cartier's information rather quickly from Peter in Albany, the mechanism underscored a problem that would only become more acute. The State Police had the Cartier family data in their Laboratory Information System, which we referred to as the Albany BEAST. This was critical information we often needed. However, we did not have direct access to it except via phone or fax until July 2002. That day in December when I was calling about James Cartier, Peter understood my urgent need. I suppose he correctly read the panic in my voice. Sometimes, though, we would have to wait a couple of days before Peter's overwhelmed staff could accommodate our requests.

After telling Patrick we had his oral swab, he seemed satisfied. Later I received a call from Jennie, who thanked me for helping her father. She said it was the most peaceful he had been since learning James died.

I met Michele Buffolino—no relation to Pat Buffolino, who was working in my laboratory—over the phone, too. Michele lost her mother, Rita Blau, on September 11. She had called on December 12 to inquire whether we had sufficient DNA to identify her mother. Michele is a terrific person. She calls me Uncle Bob. She came to our regularly scheduled family meetings and listened intently to our updates. She always asked, "Did you find Mommy?"

It always broke my heart, and I felt so inadequate. When we received new data, I always checked to see if we had found Rita. We never did.

15 AN IMPORTANT ROLE FOR METADATA

In early October, I suspected we had problems with the cataloging of the family samples at the Family Assistance Center. I hoped my suspicions were wrong. However, if the State Police cataloging system was badly flawed, we ran a huge risk of assigning the wrong name to a DM and returning remains to the wrong family.

Metadata is non-DNA data, information needed to assign family names to DMs. It is as critical to the overall identification process as the DNA. Corrupt metadata corrupts the entire process. If we could not sort out the metadata associated with, say, a toothbrush, then I had a major problem. If the DNA profile from a toothbrush matched a DM, but the information linking that toothbrush to a family was incorrect, I might return someone's remains to the wrong family.

When families took their loved ones' personal effects and kinship swabs to the Family Assistance Center, the NYPD collected them, cataloged them, and put them into labeled, sealed bags. These were taken to the New York State Police Forensic Investigation Center in Albany. The data associated with these samples, the information that linked a missing person to a family, went with the samples. Neither the data nor the personal effects and kinship swabs went to the OCME in the city.

How did the identification process work?

The process turned out to be an evolving one. We obtained a DNA profile from a DM recovered from the World Trade Center site. Then we compared that DNA profile with a DNA profile obtained from a personal effect, such as a toothbrush from a victim, that the family had given to the New York City Police Department at Pier 94.

Even though we could have matched the two DNA profiles, the DM still would not have a name. When we make that match, all the information my laboratory had was a State Police laboratory–assigned number associated with the toothbrush. This coded number was linked to another number. To get the family name, we had to call Peter Wistort, who would look up the toothbrush information and then fax us the DNA profile from the toothbrush as well as the accompanying family information. My laboratory would confirm Peter's information by cross-checking his information with what we had on file. Also, we manually compared the STR profiles from both the DM and the toothbrush.

On the surface, collecting family samples and personal effects seemed simple enough. Families went to the Family Assistance Centers, where they were interviewed by NYPD personnel. They filled out the seven-page questionnaire (Victim Identification Profile designed by DMORT) and then gave samples, either then or during subsequent visits. Several collection centers surfaced in the ensuing months after September 11. The first was at NYU Medical Center next to the OCME headquarters building, then at an armory on 26th Street, and finally at Pier 94 on the west side of Manhattan.

The New York City Police Department assigned each missing person a P number for those families that came to the Family Assistance Centers, or a T number if the family phoned in the information. A family might have both P and T numbers. The NYPD also assigned a DNA collection number if the family brought personal effects or gave family samples, such as oral swabs. The DNA collection number was simply a number. It had no prefix or suffix.

A family coming to one of the Family Assistance Centers with personal effects should have walked away with a P number and, ideally, a DNA collection number. If the family had previously called or called later with information, they should also have had a T number.

If a second family member came to the Family Assistance Center, say, at a different time, to provide an oral swab, they would be given yet another DNA collection number. To complicate an already confusing situation, if the family inadvertently brought samples directly to the OCME, which happened in the period right after the attacks, the OCME assigned an FR number.

In reality, families made multiple visits to various collection centers. It is understandable that the process was confusing to both the families and to those collecting the specimens. Each visit generated at least one number.

How confusing was it?

The Cartier family had two P numbers, a T number, an FR number, and five DNA collection numbers. Multiply this single family by thousands, and the resulting confusion was mind-numbing.

There were even more numbers. In fact, the World Trade Center effort became a numbers confetti. The New York City Police Department transported the family samples to the New York State Police Forensic Investigation Center in Albany, where they received yet another number, a WDI number, one for each delivery. A family could have more than one WDI number; the Cartier family had three.

In the scenario I described matching a DNA profile from a DM to a toothbrush. In reality, we were matching the DNA profile of the DM to yet another number, an SP number. The SP number was a New York State Police number assigned to the DNA extract of a specific personal effect; in this instance, the toothbrush. These numbers had a specified format: SP–XXXXX–XX, which might be SP–00095–16. Translation: the 95 refers to a specific batch of DNA extracts, and the 16 refers to the position of the sample in a microtiter plate. Even knowing this information was not sufficient to give the DNA profile on the toothbrush a name. The tracking software, the BEAST maintained in Albany by the New York State Police, cross-referenced, that is, linked a WDI number or multiple WDI numbers to each SP number, such that pairing the SP number with the WDI number provided the name.

After making a match, Elaine Mar, the supervisor of the OCME second-floor World Trade Center DNA identification unit, would call the New York State Police and give them the matching SP number. Then she would have to wait until Peter Wistort faxed the cross-referenced WDI number with the name of the missing person.

The process really was simple in concept, and once everyone understood how it worked, it was easy enough to implement, assuming, of course, that the numbers were correct. This turned out to be a huge assumption.

I met Mike Hennessey on September 28 at the Saturday meeting with Howard Cash when he brought his GeneCodes group to New York. Mike works for Howard and has an MBA from the University of Michigan Business School. Slightly short-statured, with dark hair, Mike's intelligent dancing brown eyes immediately catch your attention. He is blessed with a mind that easily distills complex information, finds the problem, and then derives a solution. His solutions often wind up in the form of flowcharts. He reveled in understanding and then explaining our complex processes to anyone, including me, who needed to see how the different work processes interacted. Once, after he and I had spent time working on a short spreadsheet project, he looked up from the computer and said, "I like to show off." I knew that already.

After learning about metadata from Dave Feldt during that Saturday meeting, I realized I needed someone to understand the metadata situation in the World Trade Center DNA process. Mike assumed that responsibility and made himself an indispensable and permanent presence in the DNA laboratory.

In those first few weeks in October, he was in and out of the lab. I never really knew where he was until he showed up. He would drop by my office and report what he had learned. He impressed me with his thoroughness. On one visit to the Fresh Kills Landfill on Staten Island, where the New York City Police Department sifted though World Trade Center site diggings for additional remains, Mike recognized what he thought might be a potential problem. In his opinion, the process itself allowed the possibility that remains might be missed. At my request, he wrote up his concerns, and I relayed them to Chuck Hirsch. A few days later, I received a phone call from an angry chief of detectives, who explained in no uncertain terms that whoever my source was, he should not have been at the landfill. He was adamant that Mike was dead wrong. Had I hit a raw nerve?

Mike kept digging and learning. He visited Pier 94 frequently, learned the inner workings of the NYPD family collection process, and made friends with the cops and DMORT volunteers. He studied everything, asked the appropriate questions, made the appropriate connections, and eventually understood exactly how family information and samples were collected and tracked. He identified where there were problems, ones that would haunt us for years.

Eventually, Mike understood the entire process better than any single person. He had a grasp on everything: the operations at the OCME, the collection at the various Family Assistance Centers, and the information flow between Pier 94, the OCME, and Albany.

Eventually, he translated this hard-won expertise into a process of checking and rechecking to ensure that, when we associated a missing person to a DM, it was correct. This is the process he developed that we called administrative review, or admin review. Knowing how valuable he had become, I put him in charge of the admin review in October 2001.

Like a chameleon, the admin review process changed as we identified new problems that needed solutions. We needed to ensure that we could recognize these problems as they occurred. Mike's flowcharts documented the changing history of the admin review, which evolved into a comprehensive and effective mechanism to ensure a family received the correct remains.

In October 2002 at a conference in Phoenix, Mike would present the admin review process publicly for the first time. He pointed out where in the New York City Police Department collection process errors occurred, mostly during the family interview phase followed by the subsequent hand entering of the data. Recording errors and inaccurate data were prevalent, and he estimated that out of the 4,500 collections, one in six had errors.

Understanding where errors occurred was critical to sorting them out. At one point, he summarized four types of problems:

One: *Lack of Match*, as in no DOB (date of birth) for the DNA donor in one record, but it is present in Victim Identification Profile, the DMORT seven-page form the victim's family filled out. This meant that the family member's date of birth did not match the one given in the Victim Identification Profile, the DMORT, seven-page questionnaire filled out by the family.

Two: *Trivial Disagreements*. These could range from typos, such as differences in dates of birth, e.g., DOB of 3/7/55 vs. 7/3/55, to alternate spellings of names like Catherine vs. Katherine. There were disagreements, such as Mary Jones vs. Mary Anderson where Jones was a victim's maiden name, that were clarified by obtaining additional information. And then there were the obvious reversals in stating biological relations like father to son, brother to sister.

Three: *Serious Disagreements*, where the problems undermined the integrity of the data. For example, a mismatch between the type of personal effect collected at Pier 94 and what was processed in Albany. Biological relationships that appeared incorrect that had no easy resolution. Instances where there were either missing or duplicate P numbers, names, case numbers, SP numbers, and DM numbers.

Four: *Gut Feel*. This was a catchall category where all the metadata matched, but it just "looked" wrong for any reason.

By late November or early December I understood the extent of the family collection problem. It was a mess. Not only were there clerical errors, which meant a nightmare for the admin review, but there were literally hundreds of families who did not have sufficient antemortem DNA from either kinship swabs or personal effects to make identifications. I discussed this with Chuck Hirsch.

At about that same time, we began meeting more or less regularly with the family groups, such as Give Your Voice. At first, we met in Mayor Giuliani's private office at City Hall. Later we met in City Hall in a room called the Committee of the Whole when the number of attendees from city agencies, such as the New York City Police Department, the OCME, the New York City Fire Department, the Office of Emergency Management, and the family representatives grew seemingly exponentially from meeting to meeting. At one point, there may have been as many as fifty people present. It was an awesome experience.

At that first meeting in Mayor Giuliani's office, Chuck and I met with the mayor and representatives of firefighters' families. They had questions about the World Trade Center rescue effort. Chuck and I were there because the families had questions about what happened to bodies coming into the OCME and also about DNA.

Most of the questions were born of ignorance, much like most of the early questions about DNA. They were also unsure of the OCME's role in the process, which ranged from remains collection at the World Trade Center site, transport to the OCME, ceremonies of the members of service versus the civilian missing, the semantics of "intact" bodies reported by the media, and, of course, the DNA process.

Most DNA questions centered on why it was taking so long to get a DNA test result. I have to admit, Mayor Giuliani was always considerate. He listened to me politely, usually asked a probing question, but rarely challenged me. I was there to provide information so that he could understand the situation. When I mentioned that a fairly large number of World Trade Center samples were not giving complete test results, his question was geared so that he understood the problem.

Of course, he demanded to know what I was doing about it. My response was to explain my degraded-DNA strategy. I never tried to mislead him or give him false hope. Actually, I purposely tried to sound more pessimistic than I felt.

At another meeting, I revealed the problem we had with missing family data. I purposely did not say publicly that much of the data was erroneous. I knew the mayor had close ties to those in the New York City Police Department, which had been responsible for setting up the family collection process, and it would have been counterproductive and unfair to point a finger. It was a problem, regardless of why or how it happened. The mayor needed to understand the implications. Even many of those families for whom we had the correct information were problematic. Many of them had not given a sufficient number of samples to make an identification. I had done a quick review and discovered that the number of affected families might total over a thousand. It was disheartening.

Though I didn't know it at the time, this is exactly what happened to James Cartier. When I had spoken to his father, Patrick, in December, we had already recovered James's remains. They were at Memorial Park at the OCME. However, we had only Patrick's DNA profile on file, which was insufficient by itself to make the identification and return James to his family.

When I mentioned the problem, I clearly read the concern on the mayor's face. For him, it had been a revelation. Again, he demanded to know what we were doing about it. Chuck mentioned setting up a DNA hotline to reach out to the families.

The last time we met in the mayor's office, I wanted to shake his hand and thank him for being such a vibrant and significant leader. I was nervous. When the meeting adjourned, most of those present snaked their way toward the door. Mayor Giuliani darted behind his desk to get something and was bending down to pick something up from the floor. I broke ranks with those filing out of the office and walked behind the mayor's desk and said, "Mayor Giuliani, I want to say it's been an honor working for you." I stuck out my hand.

The mayor stood up, seemingly a bit stunned. He stared at me for just a second, then smiled and grasped my hand, shaking it, and said, "You're doing a great job."

My first thought was that I wished the entire lab staff could have heard his words. His remark was really meant for them.

With Mike Hennessey spearheading the admin review, I felt confident we were assigning the correct names to the DMs. To show how complicated even a simple process like proving that a toothbrush came from the proper missing person can be, I have taken one of Mike's reports, removed any identifying information, and paraphrased it below.

COMMENTS

DNA Donor is "Westchester County/D.A." MLI Carla De-Vito looked into the matter: Westchester County DA Office acted as a collection site and a New York City Police Department Sgt from the Bronx Task Force is in her notes. It confirms that the deceased's brother submitted personal effects. He was staying with his sister, whose husband is also missing.

The Pier 94 spreadsheet shows only two collections at the Westchester County DA Office, both on Sept. 24, 2001. Two New York City Police Department officers witnessed both collections. The deceased's items were two toothbrushes (which match each other), two nail clippers, and a razor (all untyped). No other collections took place.

The husband's collection was a toothbrush. Later his parents gave swabs after they had been contacted via the hotline. The swabs do not show a relationship to any of the effects collected at Westchester for either victim. This shows that the husband's personal effect was not switched with the deceased's at the Westchester office.

One DM was identified as the deceased's by dental X-ray, but its profile is negative in MFISys. A review of the raw data for BodePlex of this DM shows uncalled peaks in the

100–400 RFU range for all eight markers and they are consistent with the personal effect for the deceased. Erik double-checked this and did not see any conflicts. The lowest stats on this profile are 1.03e+8 in the Caucasian population. In addition, this DM came into triage with the deceased's wallet in the pants pocket.

The P number for the deceased is unique to this victim and there are no other victims with the surname. In addition, the missing persons log number used for the DNA collection at Westchester is the same number in the deceased's police log filed by his sister.

SUMMARY

We have several identifiers that are unique to the deceased: P number, MPS number, and surname.

The DA collection site is a closed population (one other victim) and we have swabs for the other victim that rule out mixture between the two cases.

The deceased's family confirms that they did donate personal effects at the Westchester DA's office.

A DM was identified as the deceased by dental and it had property belonging to the deceased. And the BodePlex of this remain matches the DNA from the personal effects at all eight markers tested, with stats no less than 1.03e+8 in any race.

Based on these factors, I would recommend accepting the profile for the toothbrush as an exemplar for the deceased.

I have always been superstitious when good things happen to me, which is why I was nervous about reporters saying nice things about me in the press. I have this strange superstition that when something good happens, it's an omen that bad must follow.

Well, our track record without mixups ended.

Our first major error occurred in April 2002. At first, everything appeared okay. We matched a DM number to an SP, the number assigned by State Police scientists to the DNA extract from a personal effect. Naturally, we were excited. All matches were exciting. After linking the family name assigned by the New York State Police to WDI number via the SP number, we would have a new identification. By April, the process had become streamlined. The earlier tedium of making phone calls followed by waiting for a fax had been swapped for an electronic link to Albany. Our lives had become much simpler.

What happened?

Remember, there were several Family Assistance Centers, where the New York City Police Department collected personal effects and family information before consolidating the Family Assistance Center operation at Pier 94. In this instance, the Pier 94 data included two P numbers—not unusual—and four DNA collection numbers.

Mike had checked the Albany records and found a fifth DNA collection number, which he interpreted as meaning that a second person's personal effects had been mixed with the first's. Searching both P numbers in all available databases, he corroborated his suspicion. One belonged to a second missing person who had been recorded with the Pier 94 records but was not among those maintained in Albany.

An exhaustive investigation showed that the fifth DNA collection sample belonged to a second deceased whose personal effects had been accidentally combined with the first missing person at Pier 94.

Mike reexamined the original packaging, investigated the people who brought the toothbrushes to Pier 94, and confirmed the mixup. The practical result was that the OCME had returned remains to the wrong family in November 2001. Mike did not find the mixup until April 2002, five months after the family received the remains.

When I told Shiya Ribowsky, it was clear that he and I would have to meet with both families. On our way to Long Island to explain the mixup to the widow, I kept searching my mind for something appropriate to say other than "I'm so sorry."

She was gracious though skeptical as we explained how the error happened. We brought the entire OCME file and showed her the data, the Albany records, and DNA records. The ordeal went as smoothly as possible, but it was extremely difficult and took its toll on both of us. Thankfully, she believed us.

The next day I asked Mike to recheck every DNA identification since September to see if there were other mixups lurking out there. We were both nervous about it because the admin reviews for most of the early identifications made in November and December 2001 had not been as rigorous as they had become by April.

16 AMERICAN AIRLINES FLIGHT 587

December 12, 2001

American Airlines 587 Bodies Identified: 265

DQ (Disaster Queens) Remains Received: 2,067

Family Samples Received: 710

Monday, November 12, was a holiday, Veterans' Day, and many in the lab decided to take the time off. The previous weeks had been hectic, chaotic, and stressful. They deserved a few hours to collect their thoughts, relax, and do something family related. Howard Baum and I were at work, still trying to fit the pieces of the World Trade Center puzzle together. I was beginning to feel like we had come a long way.

The first Kinship and Data Analysis Panel in October had given us statistical guidelines for making identifications. I had hired Gene Codes Forensics to write software that would give us the ability to link mtDNA and STR data (though that project would grow into a much more complex exercise). We were already using WTC CODIS to make direct matches to personal effects. Our borrowed laboratory information system, the BEAST, was tracking DMs coming to the lab, which gave me a much better feeling about not mixing up DMs. Thanks to Lydia's group, accessioning was running smoothly. The lab had also produced approximately 900 DNA profiles on DM tissues. Actually, I was feeling a bit cocky.

I don't recall the precise time, but I would guess it happened sometime between 9:00 A.M. and 11:00 A.M. The radio was on. That's when I heard it. An airplane had crashed in Queens!

The bastards did it again! I thought.

Then I thought, It has to be a mistake. Then I thought . . . prayed. Maybe the plane actually crashed in Nassau County. Maybe it's someone else's problem. I had enough headaches of my own. Let someone else do it.

I was not that lucky.

The plane crashed in Rockaway, Queens, with more than two hundred on board. The final tally would be two hundred sixty-five, a combination of those on the plane and on the ground. It turned out to be the largest airliner crash in North American history, and the fourth-largest mass fatality in the country's history; only the World Trade Center, the 1906 San Francisco earthquake, and the 1904 sinking of the *General Slocum* topped it.

Howard and I looked at each other in silence, dumbfounded. After listening to a commentator describe where it crashed, I was hoping I really hadn't heard that the crash was in Queens. I thought for a moment, then said, "Hey, we can do this ourselves."

Howard agreed.

Had we lost our minds? We already had the largest mass disaster in the history of the United States. Was I really seriously considering handling an airline crash?

The DNA work associated with an airliner crash is a huge project that can completely overwhelm a laboratory. The Swissair crash had 229 aboard, for which the Royal Canadian Mounted Police analyzed more than 1,200 samples. I thought about having the work sent to the Armed Forces DNA Identification Laboratory, but they were still working on the Pentagon and Pennsylvania crashes. What about the FBI? No!

Perhaps the strain of the World Trade Center was getting to me or maybe I simply had confidence in my staff. I'm not sure which, but I felt we could handle it.

Then I began having second thoughts. Did I really want to get involved? That Howard agreed without hesitating or reminding me of problems we would face was, in itself, interesting. It was also reassuring. I made the decision.

The OCME had settled into a mass-fatality routine and so had the lab. Remains from World Trade Center victims were coming in constantly. Adding new autopsy tables and reassigning ME shifts was not a big deal. Accessioning the World Trade Center remains in the lab had also become routine. Adding another numbering system to the BEAST would not be a problem. Lydia's group could handle it.

Ralph came to me shortly after we learned of the crash and asked if he could go to the scene. I knew there was a huge fire, and the memory of how empty and awful I felt when I thought I had lost him and MESATT after the first World Trade Center tower fell clawed into my consciousness. I reminded him of that. He stared at me a moment, then said, "I have to go."

"How will you get there?"

"I'll take my Jeep."

Although I tried to understand what he was feeling, I realized this was something he had to do. It was sort of like climbing back on the horse after it bucks you off. Still, I was afraid he would get hurt. "Just be careful."

I didn't realize it until later, but his asking had been courtesy. He had already talked to Dave Schomburg and was ready to bolt.

"Stay in touch," I said, as he left the office.

Chuck Hirsch and I had a short conversation about alternatives, much like we did after the World Trade Center attacks. He wanted to handle the DNA typing and make the identifications in-house. There was nothing else to discuss.

"Howard and I already decided we can do it," I said.

In actuality, we ended up not doing all the DNA typing in-house. I was still against analyzing bones in the laboratory, so Lydia sent 243 bones to Bode.

I left Chuck's office feeling okay about assuming control over the

American Airlines 587 DNA identification effort. Just thinking about looking for another group of laboratories to outsource the effort to and then managing it was draining. How much could I handle? I thought that outsourcing would only complicate the situation.

How many samples would we eventually receive? Based on the number the Royal Canadian Mounted Police received in the Swissair crash, I expected a relatively small number, perhaps 1,500 to 2,000. I was wrong. My estimate did not include the family samples. Analyzing the samples would not be easy, considering that we still had criminal casework, too.

Then Chuck Hirsch shocked me. "Do you think you can get the DNA work done within a week after the last autopsy?"

I was stunned. Was he serious? It seemed unfair to ask so much of a laboratory that was completely immersed in the World Trade Center work.

"Maybe," I said, knowing it would take weeks to recover the bodies and to complete the autopsies. I did not argue because I thought we might actually do it.

To differentiate them from World Trade Center remains, the OCME assigned the American Airlines Flight 587 remains DQ (Disaster Queens) numbers to differentiate them from DM remains. The DQ remains began arriving in the lab that evening, the first samples being blood.

Lydia's disaster group accessioned them alongside the World Trade Center remains. We did the World Trade Center and American Airlines Flight 587 work simultaneously, neither taking precedence, neither hindering the work of the other. Once, I even thought the lab might have a permanent mission to work on mass-fatality events. It seemed almost surreal.

We adapted quickly, and the entire lab pulled together once again. I cannot express how proud I am of these dedicated young people. We had two disasters of historic proportions yet had not missed a beat. We never stopped working on homicides. Our routine work, such as sexual assaults, continued unabated.

Chuck's decision to process the DQ remains in-house sent us on an analytical path different than the one chosen for the World Trade Center. The next day, I met with Howard Baum, Marie Samples, Pat Buffolino, Karen Dooling, and Mecki Prinz, my senior management staff.

For directly matching DNA profiles, we decided against CODIS. Instead, we chose a Quattro Pro spreadsheet. Mecki and Marie assumed that burden because Howard was gone during that first week for a Jewish holiday. Mecki and Marie checked the STR data and entered them into the spreadsheet. When Howard returned, he programmed the spreadsheet to hold the American Airlines Flight 587 data and also added macros so that he could make direct matches. Previously, he had designed our local OCME DNA database, which we call Linkage and which we use routinely for searching crime scene profiles for matches before putting them into CODIS.

Mecki wrote to the staff on November 13, explaining that the World Trade Center disaster team would accession all American Airlines Flight 587 remains and World Trade Center remains and extract the DNA from the tissues, while regular casework rotations would work on quantifications and STR typing. We would process the American Airlines Flight 587 remains separately from the family kinship swabs and the personal effects.

Marie and Mecki reviewed the American Airlines Flight 587 data for accuracy and validity before handing them off to Howard, who would input them into the spreadsheet for matching. As the weeks wore on, the plastic magnetic letter box sticking on Howard's office door, which we use to transfer mail and data among lab staff, had become so heavy that it often sagged or even slid to the floor under the weight of American Airlines Flight 587 STR data.

Howard spent hours entering the data and searching it for matches, much of it on the weekends. He and his family deserve huge kudos for giving up their valuable time so that the families of the American Airlines Flight 587 victims could have their loved ones returned.

As I mentioned, Lydia's group extracted the DNA from the tissues using the Promega IQ system, which we had recently used to complete the validation on the World Trade Center work. On November 12, Lydia's e-mail explained the process and concluded by writing, "We need help with the midnight to 8:00 A.M. shifts." This was the first clue that this would not be a slam dunk.

Mark Desire organized the American Airlines Flight 587 family samples project. Jaded by delays in the World Trade Center work, I wanted us to have the ability to match their DNA profiles to the DQ DNA profiles as soon as the data were available.

The regular OCME DNA lab staff did the family sample work. Mark Desire set up four working evidence exam tables at our Bellevue evidence examination laboratory, which is four blocks away from our main DNA laboratory. Criminalists examined the family samples, chose the candidate sample that would give a complete DNA profile, put the samples into labeled tubes, and transported them—walked them four blocks down the street—to the DNA lab. Other criminalists extracted the DNA, treating these as routine cases. The DNA extracts went through the normal DNA STR-typing process.

Eventually, Mark would supervise the World Trade Center family sample accessioning and processing after Tom Brondolo and Shiya set up the DNA hotline in January 2002.

I first met Mark when he came to my laboratory for a job interview in the summer of 1997. His recent master's degree in molecular biology made him a prime candidate to work in the lab, so my concern wasn't so much for his scientific ability, which I did not doubt. But Mark is a husky, muscular guy, so I was more interested in whether he played softball. He did, so I hired him.

Mark was with MESATT at the World Trade Center site on September 11 and almost died when the first tower collapsed.

Although we had put into motion a plan to process American Airlines Flight 587 samples and to obtain DNA profiles from the remains and from the family samples, I had the same problem I had with the World Trade Center effort. I would have DNA profiles but could not make identifications.

Well, that's not entirely true. Howard's spreadsheet enabled us to make direct matches to personal effects, but I had no way to make kinship identifications, which would become the most prevalent method for making identifications from American Airlines Flight 587 remains. Many of the family structures, the pedigrees, of those who died in the crash were extremely complex because entire families perished when the plane crashed. We didn't know this until we began receiving information from an American Airlines liaison with the families, information passed on to the laboratory by the medico-legal investigators under Shiya Ribowsky's direction. For these families, identifications made by direct comparison of the DQ samples to personal effects would not be possible. Those samples did not exist.

Shiya, deputy director of Medicolegal Investigations, was responsible for reporting identifications to the New York City Police Department, which would inform the families. Before the World Trade Center disaster and the plane crash, medicolegal investigators at the OCME were responsible for investigating suspicious death crime scenes. Their role was to determine whether a death would become the responsibility of the medical examiner. I had had little interaction with them before the American Airlines Flight 587 crash. However, the crash changed that because we needed each other to make the correct identifications.

I'd known Shiya for several years, mostly as an acquaintance as in, "How're ya doin'." He is dedicated and compassionate, which made him the perfect intermediary between the OCME and both the American Airlines and World Trade Center families.

He had the unenviable responsibility of notifying the families and rectifying misidentifications. It was an emotionally draining task. On one occasion, a clerical error caused a misidentification, and he had to travel to the Dominican Republic to tell a family that he had to take remains away. His reward for doing the right thing and being honest was spit in the face.

The relationship between the medical legal investigators and the DNA laboratory grew steadily because of the American Airlines Flight 587 work. The medicolegal investigators received their investigative information, such as family relationships and buccal swabs, from an American Airlines representative assigned to the OCME. From this, they formed "hunches" and relayed them to either Mecki Prinz, me, or Howard Baum. Mecki and I checked DNAView for kinship matches while Howard checked his spreadsheet for direct matches to personal effects. In several instances, their "hunches" proved prophetic and saved us a lot of time.

In mid-November, Charles Brenner thought DNAView was ready for kinship identifications. Mecki sent him the first set of American Airlines Flight 587 data, including family samples, and Charles ran it through the program's new Disaster Screen function. It worked beautifully. The next day, he sent us a list of potential kinship identifications, which we started investigating.

Near the end of November, Charles installed DNAView on our computers and gave us a kinship analysis lesson. It propelled us forward, not only for the American Airlines Flight 587 but also for subsequent World Trade Center identifications.

Finding and confirming the identifications, whether they occur by kinship analysis or by direct matching to personal effects, are time consuming and tedious. DNAView is clunky and counterintuitive. Howard's spreadsheet required extensive cutting and pasting to find the direct matches.

The American Airlines Flight 587 and World Trade Center identifications came in bunches. The only difference between the two disasters, with respect to making direct identifications to personal effects, is that for the World Trade Center we were using the FBI's CODIS. For the American Airlines Flight 587, we used Howard's spreadsheet. We used DNAView for both.

On December 12, exactly one month to the day after American Airlines Flight 587 crashed, we identified the 265th missing person. We had made just the one error, a clerical mistake that I made that sent remains to the wrong family. And which Shiya rectified.

• • •

We completed the American Airlines Flight 587 identifications in record time. Although there were still human fragments we had to repatriate, we completed the identification work only two weeks late, according to Chuck's time line. My staff deserves medals for their perseverance, dedication, and compassion.

On the second anniversary of the American Airlines Flight 587 crash, Chuck, Shiya, and I would attend the memorial service at the crash site in Queens. The day was cold and rainy. I did not attend the first anniversary, but Shiya said that the weather for it was exactly the same. My feet were wet and cold. Shivers kept coursing through my body. It was eerie.

We stood in the back of the crowd and watched people hand out white roses, a symbol of eternity. The Red Cross was giving people clear plastic ponchos, so they could stay dry, and Kleenex to those who were crying. We listened to Mayor Michael Bloomberg deliver a well-thought-out, politically correct speech. A choir sang several moving songs, and a young woman read a letter in Spanish that she had received from her mother, a letter written just before she had boarded the plane. I understood only a few of the words, but the letter's intent was clear. When she finished, she broke down.

It was a sad day.

17 EMPHASIS

December 31, 2001

DNA Identifications: 99

Remains Received: 12,360

Personal Effects at NYSP: 3,447

My October 8, 2001, letter to Howard Cash had officially asked Gene Codes Forensics to write DNA-matching software for the World Trade Center DNA effort.

I was concerned with mtDNA data and how to combine it with STR data to make matches. I was still secretly praying the FBI would upgrade CODIS. I wanted CODIS to be my first-line matching software, but I needed Gene Codes Forensics to be my backup.

Eventually, the city established a contract with Gene Codes Forensics to write the program, which would become MFISys. I wanted the program to be available to other public laboratories, so that no one would have to walk in my shoes again. However, my letter was not an "official" contract, which meant that MFISys would be a commercial product and would not be available to other public laboratories unless they purchased it. This would become a sticking point in the future.

When I wrote the letter, I knew I was taking a chance. I realized the FBI would never bring CODIS to the point where it would do what I needed. Here was my gamble: Gene Codes had written only a single molecular biology computer program, Sequencher. I had no guarantee they could write the program I needed. This entire project was a leap of faith, perhaps blind faith, on my part.

It is also fair to say that my expectations were exaggerated. I did not have the foggiest idea how long it would take to write the program. Naïvely, I expected a finished product, perhaps not polished, within a couple of weeks.

But I had no choice. I had to wait to see what Gene Codes Forensics would deliver.

Finally, Howard Cash called. He wanted to show us his first ideas. He came into the lab near the end of November. Late that afternoon, Howard Baum, Mecki Prinz, Karen Dooling, and I watched intently while Howard Cash demonstrated the features of a program he was calling MFISys—pronounced *emphasis*—which stood for Mass Fatality Identification System. Early on, I affectionately called it the "Mighty Fine Identification System."

Howard demonstrated the program's features, but much to my surprise, it was not a working program. He was showing us mocked-up screen shots of a program still under development. I mistakenly thought he had brought a finished program. Once again, I had to wait.

My impatience was related to the reams of data on paper that CODIS continually spit out for Karen and her ID group. They waded through piles in order to find DM and personal effects matches. The CODIS approach was tedious and slow, and each time they received new data, I was more convinced this was not the best way to do this work. We would never get to the end of this project unless we had something more efficient.

The first version of MFISys, version 0.1, arrived on December 13. Howard Cash walked Howard Baum, Karen Dooling, and me through its features—the real program. As the features came alive on the screen, I actually had goose bumps. I could not believe what I was seeing, and my enthusiasm grew with each screen shot. I immediately began to feel at ease. I realized I had made the correct decision to work with Gene Codes Forensics and not the FBI. Within a little over two months, Howard Cash's company had taken nothing more than the concepts we had discussed and turned them into something more appropriate for identifying human remains than CODIS. This was the first version, so more would come. I felt great.

By having Gene Codes Forensics under contract, I could direct MFISys's development and ensure the company tailored it to our requirements. This turned out to be important, because our needs changed dramatically and often over those first few months.

Over time, however, the contract became a problem. Gene Codes burned through the funds quicker than expected, and although the proper people knew about it, the contract was not extended expeditiously, and Gene Codes Forensics walked off the job, twice.

But as MFISys unfolded, the pieces of the World Trade Center puzzle finally began falling into place. That first version made all the difference in my expectation for successfully finishing the work.

During those first few months, I silently measured our success against the forensic dentists because, to me, although they were nice people, they were cocksure that forensic dentistry was the rosetta stone for mass-fatality human identification. Forensic dentistry, or odontology, has become the workhorse identification method for mass-fatality incidents. Officials collect dental records, X-rays, of the missing people from the families. Then the dentist compares the teeth from the jaw of a recovered person in the mass-fatality incident against the known dental records of the person. If they match, there is an identification. And so far, it had been, with the DNA effort having produced only 99 identifications, far fewer than the dentists' 157 at December's end. I had always been certain that time would reverse the situation. In December, however, I acutely felt the competition and the pressure.

PART II
MORE THAN SCIENCE

18 2002: A NEW YEAR

January 31, 2002

Missing Identified: 666

DNA identifications: 132

The new year began unceremoniously. I was at home alone, while my wife, Fran, was caring for her mother in a Tampa, Florida, hospital. It was the first time in nineteen years we celebrated New Year's apart. I felt badly for her. She had lost her father in 1998, still hadn't gotten over that, and I knew that having her mother so sick had to be particularly difficult. I was enjoying the solitude because it gave me the opportunity to mull over our World Trade Center work, reflect on the progress we had made and where we had yet to go. More important, it was a time to relax and to put the pieces of my mind back into some semblance of order.

Around six o'clock on New Year's Eve, I found myself standing in front of the TV sipping a glass of Merlot. The news was on, but I was not really paying attention. I wasn't exactly hungry, but my mind was halfway between a half-eaten, three-day-old bucket of Kentucky Fried Chicken still lurking in the refrigerator and deciding what else to feed myself. Fran and I always made a point of eating out on New Year's Eve, but I did not relish the thought of sitting alone in a restaurant watching others enjoy themselves.

My mind refused to let go of the World Trade Center work. I was thrilled that we finally had resources in place to make identifications, and I believed I had started the process whereby we might begin to identify those whose remains were badly compromised, especially those that could not be identified only by DNA.

The data was now flowing into the second-floor DNA identification unit biweekly, and the database was beginning to grow nicely. We were receiving Myriad's STR profiles, Bode was producing them from World Trade Center bones exactly as promised, and my laboratory was extracting DNA from World Trade Center tissues and sending the extracts to Bode. Even those STR profiles were beginning to show up in the DNA management software being written by Gene Codes Forensics, MFISys.

The State Police laboratory in Albany was still sending DNA extracts of personal effects to Myriad, and those STR profiles were showing up in MFISys, too. The analytical process was taking on a life of its own. Soon, I expected, we would reach that critical mass of data where identifications would come more easily.

There were times in November and December when I was helplessly frustrated. Identifications were only trickling in. I guess this frustrated Chuck Hirsch, too. To an outside observer, our MFISys database of hundreds of profiles might have seemed like a lot, but given the number of remains that still needed DNA typing, those that had given only partial results, and the family and personal effects that still needed typing, I knew we needed a whole lot more before we would see a regular flow of identifications. We really did not begin making steady direct identifications—matching World Trade Center site DNA profiles to personal effects—until Howard Cash delivered the first version of MFISys on December 13.

On Sunday, January 6, 2002, Karen Dooling wrote to the lab that we had twenty new identifications waiting in the wings. Great news! Although we had a minor problem with the network and couldn't get these to Shiya's medicolegal investigators, I felt like we were finally pulling our weight. It was about time.

I recognized the hidden problems lurking within the family information collected at the Family Assistance Centers, so I was wary of each new identification because these issues could threaten the entire process. Data was missing, and I hoped it resided in Albany. The data that I had access to at the OCME was only a snapshot of what the state police had inventoried.

Peter Wistort, the state police CODIS manager, and his staff were always wonderful about getting us what we needed, but the system often riled me to the point of exhaustion. My staff was tired of having to call Albany in order to obtain family data and, while the system worked, it was slow. I did not have the control I needed. The scientists at the state police lab were terrific and exacting with their work, but I wanted the information at my fingertips when I needed it.

There also seemed to be a multitude of confounding odds and ends. Months after September 11 we still did not have a reliable manifest of the missing. It amazed me that the final tabulation of those who had died remained elusive. Shiya and Tom Brondolo had been working to finalize the manifest. Their goal was to assign each missing person a single number. Ideally, this would be a sequential one for each missing person and would incorporate all known information about each family. They called this number the RM, or reported missing number, which Shiya would not finalize until January 2004, when the official tally became 2,749.

Shiya used his connections in the mayor's office, the New York City Police Department missing persons unit, and the city's law department to finalize the list. When I first found out about the RM number idea, I thought it was just another number heaped atop an already bloated nomenclature nightmare. I was both right and wrong. It certainly was another number, and while the DNA effort did not necessarily require RM numbers, it eventually helped organize our work. The tricky part was for the new RM numbers to reconcile with Albany's WDI numbers, the P and T numbers the New York City Police Department assigned to families, DNA collection numbers, and the various other numbers assigned along the way.

The RM number remained elusive for so long because, aside from families who never contacted the OCME, there were the fraud cases that had to be investigated. Although there were only forty, I found even that number appalling. I cannot grasp how anyone with a conscience or a love of America would deliberately falsify someone's death just to collect insurance money. Interestingly, none of the death certificates issued by judicial decree for those whose remains were not recovered were found to be fraudulent, since a judge had to be convinced that someone's loved one really had been at the World Trade Center and had died there.

Mass-fatality events are typically classified broadly as either open or closed systems. Since we did not have a manifest, the World Trade Center work was known as an open system. The American Airlines Flight 587 crash was different. It was a closed system because we had a passenger list.

Mike Hennessey of Gene Codes Forensics was bringing me a growing number of snippets suggesting the metadata problems were far from isolated events. The WDI (World Trade Center DNA Identification) numbers assigned to each family by the State Police, supposedly one per family, seemed hopelessly redundant. This problem was not created by the state police, but was more the reality of how the New York City Police Department collected the family samples, which reflected how and when the families brought them to the Family Assistance Centers. Although I did not know about it before these problems surfaced on my radar, Shiya and the medicolegal investigators independently realized there were metadata problems. They, too, found themselves wrestling with the conflicting and redundant information.

I had to make sense of the growing mess. I asked the National Institute of Justice contractor, whom I had asked to be the World Trade Center program manager, Steve Niezgoda, to correlate the data we had in New York City with what they had in Albany. Steve immediately recognized several issues we had to resolve: conflicting data, missing data, and erroneous family data. He convened a series of weekly logistics meetings that alternated between Albany and New York City.

John Snyder is one of the more organized people I have ever met. When it was his turn to update his work, he delved into a lengthy discussion, sparing no details. During a conference call with my staff, the state police, and the folks at the National Institute of Justice, John remarked that the World Trade Center DNA effort was like "building the plane while we're flying it," a thought Shiya also remembered having. They were right. In September 2001, we had nothing. By January 2002, we had a plan and a rudimentary process in place, although we had a ton of work yet to do and a myriad of problems to solve.

Although John had been hired originally by the state police to work on their recent BEAST acquisition, the OCME needed someone who understood the Albany BEAST where the family data was housed. We wanted to connect the Albany system to the OCME BEAST, which housed all the World Trade Center DNA data on remains. A T1 line was to be set up between the two agencies so they could share data. John and Raju Venkataram, the OCME director of management information systems, worked together, but bureaucratic delays stalled it until later in 2002. These delays occurred frequently because, in my opinion, government employees are typically overextended and can't work on projects until they appear to be crisis-bound.

On January 8, 2002, Steve called the third in the series of his logistics meetings. Tom Brondolo and his IT staff, Shiya, Steve, and I represented the OCME. Mark Dale, Barry Duceman, and John Snyder came from the state police. This meeting initiated the process of trying to make sense of the erroneous New York City Police Department–collected state police family data. John Snyder brought two blue three-ring binders filled with the Albany BEAST family information. These lovingly became known as the Albany Blue Books. They contained the existing family data for those families whose personal effects had been collected by the NYPD. The personal effects had been taken to the state police, who categorized them. This was my first glimpse at anyone's idea of a missing-persons list.

A quick glance at the data frightened me. It was full of seemingly hopeless redundancies, a product of the Family Assistance Center collection process.

Though error-plagued, simply having the Blue Books made life easier. I finally had the bulk of the Albany BEAST data at my fingertips. It was a godsend because I could interact with the families immediately instead of acting as a go-between with the state police. Unfortunately, families that had not given samples at the family collection centers were not included in the Blue Books, which meant the books were not a comprehensive snapshot of all the families who had lost loved ones. The books had approximately 3,400 entries.

John had the unenviable task of reconciling the Albany Blue Book data, distilling it down to create a single list of missing people, and then reconciling this information with Shiya's RM numbers. It was a daunting task. After weeks of work sorting and analyzing, he ended up with more than 700 families whose files had major administrative problems. In time, he managed to whittle this number to approximately 200 seemingly unresolvable cases. John had been working from Albany and could go no further. Mike Hennessey, Carole Meyers, and a medicolegal investigator, Joanne Feliciano, attacked the problem from the OCME side. Over a long weekend, they managed to resolve all but a couple of dozen.

The redundant and erroneous information in the Blue Books highlighted a critical need. We needed a reliable way to interact with the families. The stark reality was that many families had no antemortem DNA, which meant their loved ones would never be returned. We needed to be proactive about it. Shiya and I discussed it and then he met with Chuck Hirsch and convinced him that we had to reach out to the families. We had to bring them into the OCME so we could collect additional antemortem DNA samples.

Mecki Prinz e-mailed me on January 3, 2002, that John Butler had completed his validation work on the Big Mini. She expected we would have everything we needed to use the Big Mini in-house by the end of January. Now I would find out whether my strategy to resurrect degraded World Trade Center samples would work. I firmly believed this would be how we would identify many of the missing.

By January 2002 the OCME staff was meeting with family members and family group representatives weekly. In addition to Chuck Hirsch and others of us at the OCME, individual family members who needed specific information, representatives of family groups, such as Give Your Voice—the family group started by the Cartier family that at one point represented more than seven hundred families—and members of the FDNY typically attended. Other government officials were usually not present, although the genesis of these meetings was at Mayor Giuliani's office, where multiple agencies—OEM, the New York City Police Department, and the FDNY—were represented. The meetings at the OCME began after one of our first meetings in the mayor's office. During the meeting, I sat beside a young woman whose husband had been a firefighter. She was confused about the DNA testing and how it was being used to identify her husband. She accepted my offer to show her my laboratory and explain the process. Unfortunately, we never identified her husband.

At the January 6 family meeting, Karen Dooling announced twenty new identifications.

The Give Your Voice Web site had spelled out a number of recurring issues that continued to gall families. Mostly, these involved statements published by the media that skirted the truth and were peripheral to the DNA effort. The families were demanding information. From the mayor, they wanted World Trade Center site tours and early notification of work stoppage—the idea was that the mayor would inform them before alerting the press. Paramount in their minds was the recurring theme of how the civilian remains were treated versus those of members of the service. At issue was the question of whether an American flag was provided to all victims at the time of recovery. Press coverage showed members of the service remains covered with an American flag. The civilians wanted their loved ones treated similarly. Other questions involved the reporting of how many remains were being recovered. This was a problem because of the semantics. Reports of bodies being recovered led the public to believe the remains were intact when, mostly, they were badly fragmented.

There were also continuing questions concerning the memorial at the World Trade Center site, a raging debate that continued even as new designs for the World Trade Center site were being unveiled.

The DNA questions were directed toward me. Thankfully, the Cartiers gave us a copy of the list before they published it on their Web site. They kindly did not want me ambushed by reporters. If I had lost a loved one on September 11 and didn't understand the science, I would have had the same questions.

How does the passage of time impact the potential of identifying a lost loved one? What is the criteria for positively confirming the identification of a victim? Can you obtain useful information with a single strand of hair for positive identification? If the hair follicle was missing or damaged, can you still obtain enough DNA for analysis? What are the precautions taken to prevent contamination of samples during collection or processing? How precise/sensitive are the methods for DNA analysis? Are the DNA methods capable of allowing discrimination between different samples in a mixture? For example, if the particular tissue samples of interest are collected with other tissues, is the current method designed to allow for adequate separation and identification of specific DNA? Who should provide DNA samples? Are all personal effects used for identification, including those that were not found on a victim? Does temperature impact DNA? I provided a DNA sample and was asked to provide a second sample because the first one did not pass testing analysis; please explain why this can happen.

Family members and reporters asked these and similar questions in varying forms to the point where I got tired of hearing them. The families' message was loud and clear. They wanted the truth, as painful as it might be.

On January 10, 2002, DNA had identified only 109 victims, less than 4 percent of the missing. We had 12,573 remains in the laboratory, with little chance of identifying most of them because we did not have enough antemortem DNA. That day, the *Daily News* ran a story emphasizing the OCME's desire to reach out to families. The article reported, "The city medical examiner's office will soon ask grieving families to provide more DNA samples to help identify World Trade Center victims . . ." The article did not mention the DNA hotline. If the reporter knew that we were planning to set up a hotline, it was not reported.

By December 12, the number of victims identified by DNA climbed to 116, with the total identified by the OCME still only 599, demonstrating the difficulty and complexity of the DNA work.

Newsday published a list, taken from the city's Web site, of the 2,189 still missing. The report said that the total number missing was 2,882, a number that would change often as Shiya continued to ascertain exactly who died. The number had changed dramatically, scaling back from an estimated 6,500 in the weeks right after September 11 before dropping below 3,000. Interestingly, the 2,882 was an OCME list, which differed from the so-called official list compiled by the New York City Police Department (2,870) and the Office of Emergency Management, which also released a daily count of victims.

The family meetings were an important vehicle for us as well as for the families because they offered an opportunity for us to brainstorm sensitive issues, including the hotline and the chapel Chuck Hirsch had constructed at Memorial Park.

With the families' blessing and Tom Brondolo's help, Shiya set up a bank of six phones and staffed them with medicolegal investigators and volunteers from my laboratory. The DNA hotline was born on Saturday, January 26, 2002. The weekend before kickoff, I gave the medicolegal investigators a *Reader's Digest* course in kinship analysis. Shiya recruited the medicolegal investigators to man the phones 24/7, which lasted until at least April 2002. It was a critical link to the families.

I was also receiving e-mails from genetic counselors who expressed a fervent desire to work with the families and the OCME staff. These professionals would have been invaluable at the Family Assistance Centers because they understand how to work with grieving families, the kinds of questions to ask, and the questions not to ask.

At the time, I was so busy I did not recognize or allow myself the time to reflect on how the stress was affecting me. I realize now that I should have thought more about it. I know my personal ability to handle stress, though high, diminishes with time and then falls precipitously. I tend to withdraw. I become introspective and quiet, preferring to be alone. I should have recognized the signs.

By January 18, 2002, Bode had received 7,120 bones and more than 3,000 tissue extracts from the sixth-floor disaster team. The company had analyzed and reported on 5,383 (28 percent). Sadly, only 2,014 samples, less than 4 percent, yielded a sufficient STR profile to make an identification. I hoped those remains having good STR profiles would yield identifications rather easily, if we had sufficient family DNA against which to make comparisons. We call this the "low-lying fruit" because picking or plucking the identifications from the "branches" was fairly easy. I had serious doubts about identifying the remainder.

Data came back to the laboratory in bunches, or data sets, because the processing of the samples at the vendor laboratories was in batches of 96. Each new data set raised new quality issues. An example illustrates the care everyone had with respect to putting STR data into World Trade Center CODIS. On January 24, Kristin Schelling, who worked for Peter Wistort at the State Police and who reviewed all the STR data, commented about failed controls. There are generally two kinds of controls: positive and negative, which are included in the DNA test with samples from the remains. Positive controls are DNA samples where we knew the STR profiles. If the STR profile developed is not correct, we know there is a problem with the test. Negative controls are "negative" and give a negative test. If the negative control gives an STR profile, again, we know there is a problem with the test. When controls failed, we had to rerun the entire set of samples. In this instance, Kristin was concerned about twenty-one samples that she suspected might have been included in the data set that had not passed quality control. These issues were top priority, and we worked to resolve them quickly.

John Hicks, the director of Forensic and Victims Services at the New York State Division of Criminal Justice Services, an arm of the governor's office, sent me inquiries from families that he had received from Lab Corp, a private forensic testing laboratory that donated its parentage sample collection centers for the families. Parentage testing is a term often used interchangeably with paternity testing. Paternity testing refers to tests used to show whether a specific man is the father of a child. Parentage is more generic and refers to testing that establishes whether someone is the parent of a child. Samples used in parentage tests are biological samples (such as buccal swabs or blood) collected at a parentage collection center.

One particularly disturbing memo asked how we had failed to find DNA in a hair sample and why we were not notifying the families directly after they sent us samples. This person was considering hiring a private company to do the testing, not realizing we were already using private labs. I thought our use of private testing laboratories had been well publicized but learned as late as September 2003 that many families had no concept of what my testing strategy had been.

Correspondence like this was tough to take. My first emotion was anger, and my impulse was to call and scold the author unmercifully. Hadn't she been reading the newspapers? Why not call me instead of sending an e-mail to a private company that had no part in the actual World Trade Center DNA testing? I had to control my frustration because I did not know who to call.

The e-mail highlighted the escalating frustration the families had with the mysterious nature of the DNA testing. Another woman wrote that after sending in a toothbrush, a hairbrush, and swabs from her loved one's parents, she had been waiting four months without news. She was angry. Her frustration was understandable, and I felt it acutely.

In this milieu, the vendor laboratories were churning out STR profiles while the OCME legal counsel was still working to finalize their city contracts. These private laboratories and consultants were working on behalf of the World Trade Center families without a contract from the city, which is unheard of. First, the city never allows vendors to work without a contract. Second, a company or private consultant would be crazy to perform work under these circumstances, since without a contract, they risk never being paid. That these companies and consultants continued to work on the World Trade Center effort speaks volumes.

In December 2001, I received a phone call from a reporter in Australia who was asking about scattered remains. I had trouble understanding what she wanted because she kept skirting the real issue. Finally, she said it. A scientist whom she had met in Australia claimed to have seen World Trade Center remains strewn outside the WTC search area.

I spoke to Dr. Richard Gould, a Brown University archaeologist. He related his belief, based on his visit to the WTC site in October 2001, that remains might be found some distance from the site.

Richard had put together a crime scene team and wanted official permission to return to New York City to check out his theory, to find what he believed would be human remains in plain view. His description of people literally crunching their way through them bothered me tremendously.

I did not know whether his theory was correct or if he had actually seen what he described. I had no reason to believe he was a crackpot or had some bizarre axe to grind. He sounded reasonable and lucid, and he had a plausible theory of how this could have happened. Also, he was an archaeologist, someone who might recognize human remains.

What if it was true? Asking Ralph Ristenbatt or someone from MESATT to retrace Richard's October steps might unearth remains from someone who might otherwise always be missing. We agreed that it would be unfortunate if someone remained unidentified because the explosion and prevailing winds had carried a small fraction of their remains beyond the World Trade Center search perimeter.

I spoke to Chuck Hirsch about Richard's wanting to bring his crime scene team to New York City. Chuck did not believe Richard would find anything, but we agreed that it would serve everyone's interests if they gave it a shot. If we did nothing, we ran the risk of having the Australian reporter publish unproven suggestions about remains lying uncollected outside the World Trade Center search area. If Richard's team found something, we might identify someone who otherwise might have remained missing forever.

On a very cold and snowy March 2, Richard led a team of seventeen volunteers—eight from Brown, four from Brooklyn College, a safety officer, a medical officer, and two Providence, Rhode Island, police officers—to New York. They met Ralph Ristenbatt, who escorted them to a roughly triangular area two blocks north of Vesey Street, which Richard had previously chosen, where they conducted a quick survey.

Ralph e-mailed me on March 4 that Richard's team recovered ten bones and bone fragments from the rear of the parking lot, which he gave to Amy Mundorff to determine whether they might be human. They weren't. Richard had suspected as much. I was rooting for them. I still thought it might be possible.

In fact, as we moved toward the beginning of 2003, we were receiving remains recovered outside the World Trade Center site search area. In one instance, workers recovered forty-three bones from a scaffold. The remains had been projected there when the planes exploded and had not been recovered immediately because the scaffold had been condemned. Richard was correct, after all.

19 FRUSTRATIONS

February 25, 2002
Missing Identified: 741
DNA Identifications: 146

In February 2002, DNA identified only sixteen people. December and January had been so promising that I thought we had turned an important corner. The number of DMs and personal effects having STR profiles had been building. What was wrong? I believed we had a mechanism to identify anyone, providing the sample gave a sufficiently complete STR profile and we had the DNA from a personal effect or kinship sample in the database. Every day I scrolled through MFISys and saw hundreds of aggregates of DNA profiles, those having the same or similar profiles, from the remains as yet unidentified. There were hundreds of orphan STR profiles from unidentified remains. Why weren't we linking these to missing persons?

In addition to not having all the remains DNA typed, we did not have a sufficient number of STR profiles from either kinship or personal effects. There were several reasons for this. The most obvious was that many families had never provided appropriate samples, which is why we established the hotline. But acquiring the samples and then DNA typing them would take time.

The second reason is that we had not yet completed STR typing on the personal effects and kinship samples. Compounding this was the disturbing fact that many of the personal effects had not yielded complete STR profiles, which meant many of them were exhibiting the same allelic dropout problems as the remains. Many gave partial profiles that would never make our statistical cutoff. A few families sent a personal effect that did not belong to their loved one. So while it might give a complete STR profile, it would never match any of the remains.

On February 2, 2002, my weekly report from Bode told me that out of the 4,774 bones reported with DNA results, only 2,352 had sufficient DNA to make identifications. Though I did not know it, this represented only about 11 percent of the remains we would eventually receive. In retrospect, we were not close to that magical critical mass of STR profiles in the database I was hoping for.

I realized that these database issues would eventually resolve themselves as we entered more and more STR profiles from World Trade Center site remains, kinship samples, and personal effects. I was also hoping that the DNA hotline would correct much of the family metadata problem.

On February 9, Steve Niezgoda sent me a memo presenting the OCME-centric view of the World Trade Center DNA software we were using. I thought I understood what software processes we had set up and what we were doing with them for our identification effort. But the complexity of the systems we had devised surprised even me. The information flow was a nasty mess. I was amazed we had allowed ourselves to get into such a precarious position.

Those of us with managerial responsibilities were extremely busy, so we were forced to solve our individual problems mostly in a vacuum. The result was predictable. Individual fixes to individual problems had led to a quagmire of overlapping, redundant, and inefficient processes. At one point, the OCME was using nine different software packages, five of which were directly related to DNA.

If someone asked me how many kin samples we had collected the previous week, I had to walk to the first-floor conference room and ask a medicolegal investigator. If someone wanted to know how many personal effect reruns—samples reanalyzed by the scientists at the

State Police Laboratory in Albany—there had been, I would either call Albany or look at what we had labeled the "Albany recuts" folder and then count the individual sheets. If my boss Chuck Hirsch wanted to know how many remains we had sent out to vendors the day before, I had to ask Lydia DeCastro. I did not know how many direct matches versus kinship matches we made or even had in the pipeline, and I had no place to go to find that information. None of the information was in a single, easily accessible location. Steve realized our ad hoc, manual system had to be revised. If software could perform much of this, it would relieve me of a huge burden.

Another burgeoning frustration concerned alternate technologies. From mtDNA, the Big Mini, and SNPs, I had a number of irons in the fire, but I was getting antsy waiting for the vendors to complete their in-house validation studies. My natural inclination was to use these technologies sooner rather than later because I wanted identifications sooner rather than later. Sometimes I just wanted to get on with it. Thankfully, I had the Kinship and Data Analysis Panel and Howard Baum protecting me from my impatient self. I did realize that waiting served everyone's—the families, the OCME, and the public—needs better. Still, it was frustrating.

Another alternate technology problem concerned how to analyze the test results. The Big Mini would produce results that we thought could be handled from within CODIS, like all the STR data. But CODIS had not been programmed to handle mtDNA or SNPs, and given its recent track record, I could not reasonably expect the FBI to upgrade it quickly enough, if ever. I was stumped what to do about it.

Steve Niezgoda believed we should treat SNPs like we did STRs, but even he was unsure whether CODIS would ever accept the data, although he thought eventually it might. I had my doubts. None of the existing DNA software packages worked with SNPs, so storing the data posed a problem. Any of the packages we were using— MFISys, DNAView, or MDKAP—would require additional programming. This would take time.

Mitochondrial DNA presented another data-handling problem. At first, the FBI suggested we might use their MitoSearch function, which was supposed to be available to us from within CODIS. It wasn't, but the reality was that I wouldn't need mitochondrial DNA immediately, so I wasn't worried yet. I had time. Based on my experiences so far, I had nagging doubts the FBI would be forthcoming with MitoSearch. As before, I had Gene Codes Forensics for my backup plan.

My original letter to Howard Cash in October 2001 specifically asked Gene Codes Forensics to include mtDNA programing. This was not exactly a flash of brilliance on my part, because the company had a track record selling DNA software. Their successful DNA program Sequencher had cornered the market. The company also had mtDNA experience with the Armed Forces DNA Identification Lab, so I felt confident that we would eventually find a way to handle the mtDNA. Getting the mitotyping data from Celera worried me more.

This was an uncertain and nerve-racking time. I still harbored nagging doubts about my ability to bring it all together. More than anything, I feared making a mistake. Steve said it in his memo titled "Goals and Philosophy," which he wrote in February 2002: "Our mission is to provide *accurate and timely* identifications, and we will always trade timeliness for accuracy."

Although my concern had always been identifications, I worried that I had forgotten something or that my personal skills or scientific inability would lead to a mess at some future time. This was becoming a very long and tedious journey, and there would be plenty of opportunities for something to go radically wrong or to uncover mistakes.

We found ourselves duplicating efforts. Someone would perform a kinship analysis and make an identification only to learn that the sample had already been reported out. Mike's group was performing admin reviews more than once, and we had no way to track whether someone was conducting an admin review or a kinship confirmation of a personal effect on another sample. Some identifications were extremely complex and required extra work. Often, two people would find out they were working on the same problem.

We were experiencing data overload, and we were overwhelmed. If someone was working on a kinship confirmation, I needed to know who it was. Information on which samples were in which processes and for how long eluded me, as did knowing who was working on what. No database told me how long we had a specific sample. I could not pinpoint who was working on which samples. This was important because the families would ask. More important, this failure eventually led to a misidentification.

Work lists loomed critical. I needed them so that we could organize our workflow. They would be a long time coming.

Concern for the families consumed a huge part of my conscious thought. Their continuing barrage of questions reinforced how important it was for them to be given the correct information. As we moved into February 2002, their queries focused on two specific areas. Many asked about the status of DNA testing with respect to their loved one. Most of this information came through the DNA hotline, but many families called me directly. It was clear that the DNA process was taking time, which made families anxious about the closing of the World Trade Center site and the landfill. They wanted reassurance that the DNA testing and the identifications would continue, so that they still had a hope that their loved one would be returned.

At family meetings and to the press, I carefully explained my plan to analyze partially degraded DNA using the Big Mini. I shared my hope that this approach would identify more people. I had to be careful not to elevate their hopes with exaggerated promises that these new technologies would work, especially since only 40 percent of the World Trade Center samples were giving usable DNA. When I mentioned the problem with degraded DNA, their sad stares and tears met my words. I never offered absolutes. All I could offer was hope and a promise to keep working.

Sometimes my words sounded hollow even to me. I had no idea whether these efforts would be successful. It was quite possible that the DNA in these badly compromised remains was not analyzable.

By the end of January 2002 and into February, the DNA hotline was receiving an unabated litany of questions. Typically, a question went something like this, "I submitted samples for DNA months ago. When I called the DNA hotline, I was told they don't have samples from me listed. What happened to them?"

The OCME prepared a written response specifically for the hotline. It was frank: "Since September 11, an enormous volume of samples were submitted to the police department and many other agencies. Some samples were not labeled properly and thus could not be used. Other samples were examined and had no extractable DNA at all. These samples were never listed."

Another common question: "After I submit the samples, how long will it take to find my loved one?"

Again, our answer was honest. "There is no guarantee we will find your loved one. DNA identification requires matching a viable DNA profile from your loved one's remains to samples you provide. With an appropriate sample we have a chance to help you; without it, we have no chance."

In mid-February, I went to Florida to help Fran bring her mother back to New Jersey to live with us. I had already made arrangements for our house to be handicap friendly, which meant putting in lifts and ramps. Fran's brother Stan did the carpentry. It was a tough time for both of them, especially for Fran because of the additional stress it caused her. It was rough enough living with a husband who was suffering from emotional stress and did not realize it, but having a disabled mother, too, seemed unfair. These meant hard times at home.

I was at the hospital in Tampa one afternoon when I received a call from Howard Cash alerting me about a sample mixup. Apparently, a bone and a tissue sample having the same core DM number had given different STR profiles, which led Howard to believe that the samples had been mixed up. The potential for mixing samples had always been there. While the news was not welcome, it was not exactly unexpected. The surprise was the messenger.

My immediate thought was, "Okay, we have a problem." My gut response said, "Why am I hearing this from Howard?" That bothered me more than the information.

Howard's staff at Gene Codes Forensic was working with the World Trade Center DNA data. And I was hearing, for the first time, that the company had been routinely running a quality check on the World Trade Center DNA data. I probably should have discussed it with Howard before, but in hindsight, this was only competent software engineering practice.

When his group discovered the discrepancy, Howard apparently felt compelled to tell someone. So he told Shiya about the potential problem, especially when I was not available, though reachable by phone. When he did call me, he neglected to tell me that Shiya was working on the problem.

Had Howard Cash alerted me to the discrepancy in the first instance, I would have conducted an investigation, which would have included resampling and reanalysis. If, after retesting, I thought we still had a problem, I would have discussed it with Shiya. Instead, after returning from Florida, I learned that Shiya had convened a joint meeting with my staff and his to discuss the mixup. This, it turns out, was the first in a series of "special projects" meetings, a joint effort between the medicolegal investigators and members of my staff. The "special projects" group worked on problem cases that required additional in-house DNA testing. Their mission was to resolve conflicts like the one Howard brought to my attention. Invariably, these were cases having discrepancies.

This particular discrepancy lingered unsolved until criminalist Erik Bieschke determined that the discrepancy was not due to commingling. The discrepancy the Gene Codes Forensics group identified was a bone with, presumably, adhering tissue. There are a number of reasons why remains having the same core DM number might give disparate DNA test results. In addition to sample mixups, another reason involves the commingling of remains. When people die together and their bodies decompose, their tissue and bone can fuse. When sampled, the tissue and the bone will give different DNA results. Unfortunately, this was a common problem we faced.

20 A CORNER TURNED

March 31, 2002

Missing Identified: 862

DNA Identifications: 208

Remarkably, by March, my days were becoming routinely hectic. I'd wake at 3:35 A.M., shower, dress, and then drive into the city, usually arriving at the OCME by 5:00 A.M. Sometimes I would have to wait in line at the Lincoln Tunnel while the Port Authority Police and National Guard checked the trucks and vans. It was unnerving and made it seem I was entering a huge, cement fort.

After crossing Manhattan, I'd arrive at the OCME and search for a parking space, something that was neither easy to locate nor guaranteed. Before September 11, the streets near the ME's office were cleaned every few days, but cars had to park on alternate sides of the street on the off chance the city's sweeper trucks would come that day. If you did not move your car, you'd likely get a parking ticket. After September 11, the city suspended street cleaning and parallel parking around the ME's office to accommodate the large number of "official" vehicles that had descended on the area. They parked perpendicular, double parked, and eventually spilled onto the sidewalks, creating mini parking lots. The doctors at Bellevue Hospital and NYU Medical Center, the cops' private cars, local residents, and those of us on the OCME staff had to duke it out for whatever spaces remained.

If the day went well, I would be back home by 9:00 P.M.

Seven months after the attacks, the scene at the OCME still seemed surreal, a constant beehive of activity. Entry into the OCME on First Avenue was restricted, a New York City Police Department barricade blocked 30th Street, and showing picture ID was required. Cops from multiple police departments throughout New York State as well as those from the city and from other cities, states, and countries milled around constantly. The Salvation Army had set up a small restaurant on the First Avenue sidewalk immediately after September 11, then moved an expanded version onto 30th Street. We called it Sal's Café, and the wonderful people who worked there served hot breakfast, lunch, and dinner until the Fresh Kills landfill closed in July 2002. It was a great place to relax, chat, and get away from the gruesome work. Send your donations. They did a terrific job.

The DMORT teams worked twelve-hour shifts twenty-four hours a day, seven days a week, ensuring a constant stream of brown-uniformed people in the lab. Mostly, they were funeral directors, and their presence was both uplifting and necessary. They worked with the sixth-floor disaster team cutting tissue DMs for DNA extraction.

After September 11, the scene around the ME's office changed dramatically from the quiet, blue-tiled nondescript building sandwiched between NYU Medical Center and Bellevue Hospital into a small, hustle-bustle city, with activity 24/7.

Sometimes when I'd arrive, I needed a cup of coffee, so I would stop at Sal's and eat breakfast before going to the second floor. The frequency of my visits to Sal's lessened after the bulges around my waistline totaled an extra twenty-five pounds. Mostly, though, I'd go directly to the second-floor DNA identification unit room and check on the new identifications from the previous day. I sat at the computer for several hours, hoping to tease out at least one new identification before 8:00 A.M. Sometimes I was confounded by complicated family pedigrees, so I would stay until I felt comfortable that I had either figured it out or needed to ask for help. There were always those days when identifications failed me, and I would go to my sixth-floor office depressed. Then there were the days when I would find them, even one, and I was euphoric. Then I could happily spend the remainder of the day working on the routine business of the city's criminal justice system. In reality, though, that rarely happened; the World Trade Center work would not allow it.

I look back on January 2002 as a breakthrough month. Shiya had established a mechanism for reaching out to the families through the DNA hotline and had begun the arduous process of sorting out exactly who was missing.

In February, the DNA workflow seemed more routine when compared to the first few months. In March I was expecting to see the fruits of our labor. More and more DNA profiles were in MFISys, and again I hoped we might finally have reached that critical mass of data.

Steve Niezgoda recognized our need to organize our processes to make the work flow more efficient. Over many dinners, he and I often talked about how the work was grudgingly becoming manageable. One night, he asked, "How many do you think we'll identify?"

At first, I did not answer. Actually, it was the second time someone had asked me that question. On the eve of the summit meeting in November 2001, a BBC reporter had asked the question. I looked at Steve and repeated what I had said then: "I guess I'd be happy if we identify fifty percent." Inside, I was thinking, How sad would that be? Months later, Steve reminded me of this when I would get depressed about how the identification process seemed to drag.

Steve worked hard to streamline our systems to maximize the number of identifications. He framed our work in terms of milestones and tried to set reasonable time lines for us to work toward. He and I often brainstormed potential target dates for specific tasks. And although I didn't realize it, he was trying to get me to buy into a series of dates that I could live with. I realized I had to steer our work in that direction, but I wasn't ready to commit myself.

On February 28, 2002, Steve handed me a piece of paper. As I read it, I looked at him and raised my eyebrows. It was a list of goals, and after each he had left a blank space. He wanted target dates. The brainstorming was over. He wanted me to commit to a time line, which I had no clue how to meet.

Meeting specific goals depended on when the World Trade Center recovery process would end. It made no sense for me to project a DNA completion date as long as remains kept coming into the lab. Most publicity was projecting the digging would end by May 30. I assumed May 30 would be the official New York City World Trade Center recovery end date. Then there was the hotline. I had no idea how long it would take to contact all the families and to receive the family samples.

I chose a date and filled in the blanks after each task. I thought we would be current on all direct-match and kinship-only identifications for which we had attempted a conventional STR analysis. This would end Phase I testing but would not include any of the alternative technologies, such as the Big Mini. I thought by June, we would have attempted STR typing on every DM sample at least once. I also speculated that we would have quality-checking procedures in place by April and that the Big Mini, mtDNA, and SNPs would go live in June.

After finishing, I stared at Steve's piece of paper. I had major doubts. How would I ever get it done? My target dates were guesses, plain and simple, but there they were, staring back at me in black and white. Were they reasonable? I had no clue.

In the end, my guesses were not far off the mark. For direct and kinship-only matches using conventional STR analysis, I was both right and wrong. Most of our easily attainable matches were completed using conventional STRs, where we had existing family information, by August 2002. The Big Mini never went online because of a sensitivity problem, and its replacement, BodePlex, did not yet exist. Mito went online shortly after the target date, and SNPs would be delayed further and not go online for another year.

On March 21, 2002, the *New York Post* reported, "Dr. Hirsch told victims' relatives at a family meeting Monday he expects DNA testing to be done eight months after all remains have been re-covered from the Trade Center rubble."

The eight-month time line came from me. It had been my best es-timate. Privately, I doubted we could really do it. It was an ambitious target, but when I made it, May 31, 2003, seemed like a long way off. I thought having committed to a time line to finish the work was pro-ductive. It gave me, my laboratory, vendors, and management "mini-missions" within the framework of the whole. Although I never shared these thoughts with anyone, these were moving targets. I was responsible for it, but most of the DNA testing was out of my hands because once the extracted samples or bones had been sent to a ven-dor laboratory, I could do little more than try to speed the process by making phone calls, which I did frequently. I often asked about spe-cific samples in the queue or why a particular shipment of data slated to go to the New York State Police, for example, was late. Sometimes I would ask to "rush" samples, but I consciously controlled my natural inclination to speed the process. I did not want to thrust these labo-ratories into the precarious position of hurrying their work, and bul-lying them would only create an error-prone, stressful situation.

It was an emotional balancing act. I keenly felt the families' angst and their desire to have their loved ones returned as soon as possible, which sometimes seemed at odds with the critical nature of ensuring that the work was done correctly.

Shiya's RM project potentially signified a radical change for the sec-ond-floor World Trade Center DNA identification unit with respect to how we identified families. Our job was to assign the correct name to a DM regardless of whether an RM number existed. Sorting through all the erroneous family data was the hard part. The RM sys-tem made the entire identification effort more manageable. And eventually it saved time by having most of the disparate family numbers incorporated under a single, composite family number. The software vendors who were programming MFISys, DNAView, and MDKAP had to do additional programming to accommodate the change to RM numbers. This was not a trivial matter and, unfortunately, it would not be the last time I forced a nomenclature change on them.

Steve addressed our burgeoning nomenclature issues in a memo dated March 2. The problem was my fault. In order to accommodate testing utilizing the various DNA technologies we were using, I had asked Lydia's sixth-floor disaster team, the New York State Police, and Bode to create multiple DNA extracts from each sample. The extracted DMs were each split into triplicates, which we called daughter extracts. Each DNA daughter extract was slated to go to a different vendor laboratory for testing. For tracking purposes and for the historical account of our work, I demanded we institute a numbering system so that anyone reviewing the data in the future would know at a glance what had happened to each remain tested. This was different than the RM system being developed by Shiya, which was a system to consolidate the missing into a single number. The nomenclature I wanted was meant to track the individual remains, regardless of whether we knew the name of the person they had come from.

Steve proposed several approaches and sent his suggestions to the software vendors, asking for their suggestions. The only caveat was that remains that had been tested already had a number that could not be changed. For example, the original tissue samples were labeled simply DM followed by a "core" number, such as DM011010. These original DMs had gone to Myriad for STR analysis. Samples labeled Bode–DM having a "core" number were bones that had been sent to Bode for STR analysis. Bode layered their numbering system on top of ours.

By insisting on knowing the analytical history of each sample, I probably made everyone's life a bit more miserable as the World Trade Center testing became more complex and the need to track more and more testing unfolded. Eventually, everything increased: the number of laboratories doing the testing, the number of samples extracted, the number of DNA testing technologies used, and the extensive redundant testing. Each sample would have its own nomenclature, sometimes several, depending on how much testing it had gone through.

By February 2002, the variety of samples, technologies, and testing formats had become so complex that Elaine's key for identifying what happened to DMs ballooned to four typed pages. It included naming conventions for DMs, quality-control samples, special-cases projects, kin samples, and personal effects.

Here's a flavor of the monster I created. Consider a DM: DM0101010. This represents an OCME tissue extract sent to Myriad. That same DM might also look like this in MFISys: BODE–DM0101010–T. This would be a sample in which the test result from Myriad was negative. It had been reextracted in my laboratory, and its DNA extract sent to Bode for reanalysis. A sample labeled BSG1–DM0101010 was a bone extracted at Bode and then sent to Orchid Cellmark in Dallas for SNP testing. Easy, huh? As the effort grew and the testing and retesting became more complicated, I found I needed Elaine's cheat sheet to figure out exactly what had happened to each sample.

When Steve sent the vendors a proposed nomenclature system and asked for their thoughts, Charles Brenner, the forensic mathematician who wrote DNAView, predictably objected and raised, for the first time, the concept of using virtual profiles to make kinship identifications. Actually, the idea applied to direct identifications as well and stemmed from the data we were receiving from badly degraded DNA. Many of the profiles were incomplete, and to assign a profile to a specific DM, it would be necessary to create a hypothetical (virtual) profile based on multiple testing of the same sample. Charles believed, correctly, that virtual profiles would become intrinsic to the success of the DNA identification work. Charles's query sent me on a mission that would define the success of the DNA identification work. It also sent me on a mission to define what a virtual profile was: how should we create them and how should we use them effectively?

A virtual profile is a single STR profile that has been constructed from two or more partial profiles, after multiple testing of the same DM or personal effect. By combining the data appropriately, it was possible to create a DNA profile composite, a virtual profile. Though each individual partial profile could not meet the Kinship and Data Analysis Panel statistical threshold, the composite could. This was critical because the original testing on DM remains did not always give complete DNA profiles, which is why I demanded additional STR testing on each DNA extract. This meant analyzing the same DNA extracts multiple times using different technologies, such as BodePlex. Sometimes the retest would come after reextracting the original remain. An example is shown in the following table.

TABLE 5. CREATING VIRTUAL PROFILES

SAMPLE NAME	GENDER	D3	D8	D13	TPOX	CSF
Virt–DM0100010	XY	15,16	13,15	8,13	8	12,13
BBB1–DM0100010	——	——	——	8,13	——	12,13
BCB1–DM0100010	XY	15,16	13,15	Neg	8	Neg
Bode–DM0100010	XY	Neg	Neg	Neg	Neg	Neg

The original testing on, say, a bone, Bode–DM0100010—the last line in the table—gave only a single STR result, the sex of the sample, a male (shaded). On the third line, the results of the Phase II—retesting using a modified reextraction technique, hence the BCB1 prefix BCB1–DM0100010—gave the same gender test result as the original testing, XY, plus three STR loci, D3, D8, and TPOX (shaded), for a total of four positive tests. A Phase III test of the same sample employed BodePlex—row two and another prefix, BBB. This test successfully yielded an additional two STR loci, D13 and CSF (shaded), both of which had been negative in the first two tests. After three rounds of testing, we had six STRs. To create the virtual profile, we combined the data into a single profile—the top line, "Virt–DM01000010"—which was our working STR profile, the one used to make a direct match to a personal effect or for kinship analysis.

The testing on this particular sample—an actual World Trade Center example with a fictitious DM number—was started in September 2002 and concluded in April 2003. This sample, even with the six STR loci identified, did not meet the statistical barrier for making matches. It still required additional analysis before it could be linked to a missing person.

We began using virtual profiles in late 2002, but before we could use them, the software had to be programmed to handle them, and I needed the Kinship and Data Analysis Panel to establish guidelines for creating them. By October 2003, virtual profiles constituted as much as 25 percent of the new identifications.

At the fourth Kinship and Data Analysis Panel meeting in New York on April 24 and 25, 2002, we addressed the issue of how to determine when two different DMs having partial profiles were pieces of the same person. This became an exercise in examining the STR profiles of two DMs by checking the loci where the DMs gave positive test results. The panel said that if the loci of a DM giving positive results gave the same STR results as another DM and the statistical rarity of these overlapping loci are equal to or greater than 10^8, the two can be considered as being pieces of the same person.

By March 2002, the hotline was generating additional World Trade Center family reference samples. These samples were being collected by medicolegal investigators at the OCME or being mailed to the OCME. Since these samples were critical to making new identifications, I did not want them subjected to the intrinsic delays of sending them to the state police for extraction, the extracts going to Myriad Genetics for DNA analysis, and the data coming to the state police for entry into World Trade Center CODIS. I decided to shortcut the process by having my laboratory do the work. I assigned Mark Desire, a supervising criminalist and a lawyer, to spearhead this effort.

On March 4, Mark wrote that 300 pieces of evidence corresponding to 87 victims had been examined in one day. It was an extraordinary effort. He did a terrific job of organizing the work, which the staff did in addition to their routine criminal casework responsibilities.

By March 5, Mike Hennessey had made the first of many flow-charts showing a decision tree for confirming matches. It had taken nearly six months of DNA testing on DMs and family samples before I felt confident we had a foolproof method for assigning the correct family name to newly identified remains. Mixups were something we had been struggling with and would continue to into the early part of 2004.

I had to be certain that none of the contract laboratories had mixed up samples during the testing process. In a March 2002 meeting with the second-floor World Trade Center DNA identification unit, Steve Niezgoda led a detailed discussion on how we could ensure that we were not making identifications from DMs that had been mixed up. We carefully examined the identification processes in place. We tackled the easy one first: the direct identification where a DM matches two personal effects. If the DM's STR profile matched a toothbrush STR profile and also a second personal-effect STR profile, say, a razor, and they met the statistical barrier, we felt confident there had been no sample mixup.

Our reasoning went something like this. The chances that two separate personal effects from the same person, which had been analyzed at separate times and had produced the same STR profile, being mixed up was too remote to be even possible. After an appropriate admin review to ensure there had been no problems with the collection of the personal effects, we reported this DM as an identification and gave the information to Shiya's group to notify the family.

In instances where there was only one personal effect, whoever worked the potential new identification put the DNA paperwork into a file labeled "Albany Confirm." When the paperwork popped up in the queue, someone would call Peter Wistort in Albany, who would retest the original personal effect. This process could take three weeks. If the STR profile of the second analysis matched the first, we had confirmed the profile. The sample had not been mixed up.

When we had only a single personal effect and kinship family samples, the admin review paperwork went into a file labeled "Kinship Confirms." The second-floor DNA identification unit analyzed the data through kinship analysis using both DNAView and MDKAP. Depending on the size of the queue, this might take a month, usually less. If the kinship analysis showed that the personal effect and/or the DM STR profile fit snugly into the family's genetic structure and also met the appropriate statistical burden, again, we had confirmed the DNA profile and had shown that there had been no mixup.

All identifications were not so simple. A son, for example, might use his father's toothbrush. This meant that the DNA on the toothbrush either did not come from the missing father or, after analysis, gave a mixture. If it was a mixture, we would not use the DNA from the toothbrush to make the identification unless we could ascertain the components of the mixture. Those situations occurred frequently enough that it was a concern, and for many of these families where we could not separate the mixture components, they would never have their loved one returned unless we could obtain another personal effect or if we had family samples with which to do a kinship analysis.

Verifying the origin of a personal effect touched every direct DNA identification. We had to be absolutely convinced that the DNA from each personal effect came from the toothbrush of the missing person. We even performed a kinship analysis on the toothbrush to prove that its DNA fit into the genetic structure of the family. In these instances, we treated the toothbrush DNA as though it were the remains of the missing person. If the kinship analysis worked, we knew the STR profile of the missing person.

Often, an STR profile did not fit the family. There were many reasons for this: the kinship sample was from the wrong family, it had been mixed up at the Family Assistance Center, the kinship relationships described by the family were not correct, the missing person was not related to the family, or the missing person was a half sibling. An important lesson learned was that family relationships were often tenuous or false. We had instances where the missing person had been adopted or had been the product of marital transgression, and a father did not know that his son or daughter was not his own. Sometimes, too, family members did not know their true relationships.

If we did not have sufficient kin samples or the kinship analysis failed because of an incorrect relationship, we asked the medical legal investigators to contact the family and request additional personal effects or kinship samples, hoping one would be available. I always felt better if we had both personal effects and kinship samples to confirm an STR profile. If one of them was incorrect, we still had a chance to make the identification.

Elaine Mar had been working on the World Trade Center effort with Karen Dooling since November 2001 before assuming the supervisory responsibilities of the second-floor World Trade Center DNA identification unit in December. She was responsible for reporting identifications to the medicolegal investigators, resolving quality-control problems, and the all-important admin review.

A young California-born woman, she's terrific, extremely bright, and a non-overbearing perfectionist. A New York oddity, to be sure. In my experience, perfectionists tend to be anal, people who normally drive me absolutely nuts. Elaine is a delight, competent, loyal, and was completely committed to the World Trade Center families. In her distinctive way, she never hesitated to let me know what she was thinking. She'd come to my office with a problem, which she would explain in exhausting detail. Then she'd wait for my response. I would offer an opinion or make a decision. If she disagreed, she would simply stare at me or look away. Not a word would pass between us until I'd say, "What's wrong?" Then we would go back to the drawing board.

On March 8, Elaine asked me to come down to the second floor. She had two new identifications and needed a kinship analysis to confirm the STR profiles, two missing brothers who might meet the statistical barrier if the kinship analysis panned out. She also had a list of twenty-three personal effects, all potential new identifications that needed someone to confirm their STR profiles. Albany would have to rerun the samples unless I did the kinship analysis. I did them gladly.

Like the rest of us, she was wrestling with the continuing and growing problem we had with redundant family numbers. They hindered our ability to relate one personal effect to another as coming from the same missing person. She noticed that, if a missing person had multiple WDI numbers (numbers assigned to a family by the state police in Albany), the missing person's relatives might be listed in two separate places: in MFISys and also at the state police. The problem was that the entries might have different WDI numbers because they were assigned at different times. We had no way to find out whether an earlier number had been assigned. If we were unable to trace these WDI numbers to the same missing person, we had an impossible identification issue. Sometimes the WDI numbers were wrong, too.

We limped into the last week of March with only about twenty identifications for the entire month, not significantly more than the sixteen we had in February. Although the number was up slightly, the work had been tedious and agonizingly slow. Sometimes it felt like we were working in a vat of molasses. I kept hoping we would soon reach a point where we would have a large enough STR database of DMs, family kin samples, and personal effects, a time when the identifications would come in bunches. But we were just inching along.

Knowing how many of the missing we had recovered was also a continuous question rattling around inside my head. Chuck Hirsch believed that many who perished had actually vaporized, a disturbing thought I consciously fought. I did not want to believe it was true although intellectually I knew it probably was.

Still, being basically an optimist, I expected a better future. I had to for myself and for my staff. If I didn't, I feared I would plunge into a bottomless emotional pit that would affect my judgment and my staff. Truthfully, the process was dragging me down.

The last week of March loomed on the horizon, and I was already wondering what April might bring. Then a miracle happened. We identified forty people.

21 RUNNING OUT OF IDENTIFICATIONS

April 30, 2002
Missing Identified: 1,107
DNA Identifications: 315

Early April. What an emotionally demanding time it was. Shiya and I delivered one World Trade Center widow some pretty awful news. Her husband's remains, which she had received in November 2001, belonged to another family. It was the most difficult time for me since the first weeks after the September 11 attacks. It didn't matter that the OCME would pay for the exhumation or that another family would be receiving additional remains. And it wasn't simply a matter of visiting her and giving her the bad news. Meeting her would be tough, but before Shiya called to make an appointment, she already knew about the mixup. Her husband's colleagues, who had insider access to the OCME, had told her that we had no intention of telling her about it. Nothing could have been further from the truth.

In September 2001, the OCME had identified a torso using personal effects and returned the remains to family 1. The left arm was missing. It was an easy, routine identification and it was absolutely correct. In November 2001, the DNA laboratory issued a report that sent a left arm to the widow of family 2, the same person to whom we had the unenviable task of delivering the heart-wrenching news. In November 2001, all seemed correct.

In January 2002, the underlying problem reared its ugly head during an admin review. Mike Hennessey noticed inconsistencies in the reference sample collection records from several families. Before January, Mike and I had suspected there might be problems based simply on a handful of cases we were working on. We really did not know how pervasive the problem was until we had the Albany Blue Books in hand, which we did not receive until January 8, 2002.

A week or so before we had the Blue Books, Peter Wistort had sent a spreadsheet containing some but not all of the Blue Book data. While searching through the information on the spreadsheet, Mike noticed the same thing that John Snyder later told us and brought it to my attention. I asked him to prepare a list of the families having these kinds of problems. Typically, he was already working on it. If someone had predicted that admin review problems would require 40 percent of my lab staff to find, document, and solve, I would not have believed them.

Mike discovered inconsistencies in the Albany collection records from family 2. We had seen situations like this before. Usually, they had not posed a problem and were solvable. The worst scenario would be if we had to take remains from a family and had nothing to give back.

In early April 2002, when this problem surfaced, the remains—which included two left arms—had already been returned to family 2 in November 2001. No one needed an STR profile to tell us that. We would have to tell both families about the mistake. A lingering question concerned the second left arm: whose was it?

I studied Mike's notes from January and saw he had jotted down family 1's name. I went downstairs to the first-floor conference room and pulled up the original photos taken of the torso given to family 1. I also looked at the photos of the left arm that had been given to family 2. The medical examiner's handwritten notes and associated diagram showed a slash across the left arm, dramatically illustrating where it had been ripped from the torso when the buildings fell. The implication was abundantly clear. I distinctly remember breaking out

into a cold sweat as I looked back and forth between the medical examiner's report and the photos. The left arm clearly belonged to the
torso given to family 1 and not to family 2. I neither needed a DNA
profile nor Amy's expertise as an anthropologist to fit them together.
The arm fit the torso like the last piece of a jigsaw puzzle.

Before we could contact the families, Shiya and I agreed we
needed to understand how and why the mixup happened. We had to
be able to explain it to both families and devise a way of ensuring that
the same mistake would never happen again.

It took nearly two weeks to investigate the problem. We learned
that someone had inadvertently placed the reference samples from
family 1 into the evidence bag containing the reference samples from
family 2. It had been a simple and understandable mistake by someone who was trying very hard to do a good job under trying circumstances. The two families had been assigned similar collection
numbers that could be easily confused.

Someone had misinterpreted a family P number for a DNA collection number. Both numbers were the same, except one had a
P prefix, the other did not. When the personal effects of both families were combined in the same evidence collection bag, family 1
became "invisible" to the state police lab in Albany, which processed both families' reference samples as though they belonged to
only family 2.

The DNA typing on the arm was correct, but the family name it
referred to, according to the state police records in Albany, was not.
No one knew until Mike uncovered the problem five months after
both families had received remains.

Shiya had the unenviable task of notifying the families. I went
with him to deliver the bad news because DNA was involved. On a
cold, sunny day, he and I drove to Long Island and met family 2's
widow. It was one of the worst moments of my life. We were delivering bad news to someone who had been told that we planned to
sweep the problem under the rug to cover it up.

We climbed three steps to the front door of the exquisitely landscaped house. The top step was small, which meant I had to stand behind Shiya while he knocked on the door. Immediately, a shiver coursed through my body, and perspiration ran down the inside of my shirt. The widow answered the door and stood in the doorway a moment, silent. It was no secret why we were there.

One of her husband's colleagues introduced us.

She was very polite, although a bit wary, and invited us into her kitchen and offered us a cup of coffee. Shiya took out his OCME folder containing her husband's paperwork, cleared his throat, and then explained why we were there. It was awkward for all of us. She listened intently, quietly, as he explained why the mixup was not the OCME's fault, but because we had the responsibility for making identifications, it fell on our shoulders. When he finished, she looked at me, which meant it was my turn. After a hesitant start, I detailed how the DNA process worked, how our analytical procedures worked, and how we ensured that DM mixups could not happen.

"How often has this happened?" she asked.

It was a great question. How we answered it would explain a lot about us and whether she should believe anything we had to say. She likely knew about a firefighter mixup that had been widely publicized in the papers. Two firefighters in the same firehouse had the same rare congenital malformation, and their remains had been sent to the wrong family. She had read about the case. But she did not know about another case because it had not been publicized. Shiya confessed to both, explaining each, sparing no details.

When he finished, she loosened up immediately. We were telling her the truth, and she knew it. She understood why after first learning about the mixup we had to determine its cause before contacting her. She confessed that a number of her friends and her husband's colleagues had been urging her to go to the newspapers.

She had waited, though, to hear our side of the story and then judge for herself before deciding how to proceed. She was gracious and fair, and I have the utmost respect for her. I only wish I could have met her and her husband under different circumstances.

Shiya and I left her house and returned to the OCME truck. I climbed into the backseat and laid my head back. Shiya turned and looked back at me. Words were not necessary. I recognized his angst and fatigue, and he mine. Although he and I had been working closely together, at that moment a bond formed between us that could never be broken. Our trip back to the OCME was an emotional roller coaster. I continually fought tears. As awful as it had been for me personally and also for her, I felt good about what we had done and prayed I would never have to go through that again.

Deep in my soul, I knew these were unanswerable prayers. I knew it would happen again. It was inevitable because many identifications had been made early in the identification process before we knew these administrative problems existed.

How many had we misidentified? It was a nagging question. Mike estimated the DNA laboratory had made 99 identifications before we instituted a formal review process. I asked him to go back and analyze each one. I had to know which ones had potential problems.

The surge in identifications, the 40 in that last week of March, continued into April. By the end of April 2002, we reported 107 new identifications. It was terrific, and new identifications filled the pipeline daily. But I knew it could not last. For starters, the statistics were telling. The identifications from dental records and fingerprints would dwindle and then stop. In April we had 16 dental identifications compared to March's 59. There was a single fingerprint identification, which I thought was remarkable given the number of months since September 11. Had anyone asked me the probability of making a fingerprint identification eight months after the attacks, I would have said, "Forget it." Not only would I have been wrong, but we actually had fingerprint identifications in October 2002 and another in late 2003 because of a new Automated Fingerprint Identification System (AFIS) that the New York City Police Department had acquired. Identifications from personal effects would be few and far between.

These facts were sobering. The vast majority of those identified after April 2002 would come by way of DNA.

With STR typing coming to an end, I expected the number of identifications to decline. I began thinking about how many we might expect to make, which brought up the concept of the number of people we had identified using DNA compared with the fundamentally different concept of the number of the missing who had been recovered. The former was really a statement of how many unique STR profiles we had in our MFISys database that had been successfully matched to a family. Figuring out the number of people we might identify was a matter of identifying the total number of unique STR profiles. The latter number, those who had been recovered, would remain unknown forever. If it was possible to figure out the number of unique STR profiles in MFISys, I thought I could speculate about a ballpark estimate when we might finish the work.

The exact number proved elusive. I had originally thought that it would be possible to sort MFISys and then count the number of stand-alone profiles. It wasn't that easy because the issue of partial STR profiles confounded the process. I did not have my first reliable data until September 2002, and it took until March 2003 when the number settled in the 1,600 range, between 54 percent to 58 percent of those who died. It was a demoralizing statistic, and at first I shared it with only Steve. If the World Trade Center work was to end at 1,600, it meant I had a time line to follow. Many identifications would come from partial DNA profiles and the process had to slow down.

I discussed the anticipated diminishing rate of identifications with Chuck Hirsch. We agreed the families should know. They had to be prepared and to understand why a decline was inevitable. Hiding our concerns might affect our hard-fought atmosphere of trust. On the flip side, I certainly had no desire to discourage them or have them give up hope.

I tendered the subject at our April 2002 family meeting. At that time, we were meeting in a conference room on the fifteenth floor of the NYU Medical Center. I had no idea how the families would take the bad news. When my turn came to speak, my internal perspiration spigot immediately switched on, drenching my shirt and making it feel cold against my skin. The uncomfortable feeling exacerbated my nervousness. Fortunately, I had worn a sports jacket. No one could see how wet my shirt had become. I walked to the whiteboard and outlined my strategy for the immediate future.

I finished and waited for an expected flurry of questions. Mostly, though, they asked me to clarify the technicalities, the science they did not understand. Now that they knew that STR testing would not carry us much further, they were curious about my plans beyond STRs. They clearly wanted the work to continue. I explained the miniplex concept and why I thought it might help. I did not mention that the Big Mini had failed. I also explained how mtDNA and SNPs might play a role in my strategy. I never misled them into believing my strategy would identify everyone.

The families understood. They knew why the number of identifications would soon slow. And they accepted that I thought it might start in August or September 2002. Unfortunately, I was right.

Every day, I relearned that managing such a large and complex project required constant scrutiny. Thankfully, I had several important professionals who kept watch over me, people who helped keep me and the analytical effort organized. Along with Steve Niezgoda, Dr. Mandy Sozer played a critically important role. Mandy was a National Institute of Justice contractor with expertise in forensic and parentage DNA analysis. She was also familiar with high-throughput systems: the robots.

She's a bright, terrific person who sports an easy, warm smile that quickly morphs into a stern, cold glare when she's not pleased; she takes her work seriously. She can be tough, which is why I sometimes affectionately referred to her as my friendly World Trade Center pit bull. When an idea popped into her head, she refused to let it go easily, a trait that made her a superb moderator for our bimonthly Kinship and Data Analysis Panel meetings.

Mandy first arrived on my World Trade Center radar in December 2001. My analytical testing scheme, though still somewhat chaotic and in its infancy, had been set in stone by then and the data were already coming back.

To recap: I had established a DNA testing program, Phase I of which was in full swing. My laboratory was extracting DNA from DM tissues and sending the extracts to Myriad in Utah. The state police laboratory in Albany was extracting DNA from the personal effects (toothbrushes, hairbrushes, et cetera) and sending these DNA extracts to Myriad. The unextracted family kin swabs were also being sent to Myriad, which was analyzing the DNA extracts from my laboratory and from the state police and also extracting and analyzing DNA from kinship swabs. The Bode Technology Group was extracting DNA from bones and analyzing them. The FBI had established a stand-alone World Trade Center CODIS network in Albany, where we housed the STR data from Myriad and Bode.

Additionally, I had worked out an arrangement with Charles Brenner, who was receiving an electronic copy of the CODIS STR data from Peter Wistort at the New York State Police. Charles created a kinship work list from within DNAView. Benoit Leclair completed his first version of his kinship analysis program, MDKAP, agreed to process the CODIS data, and sent us his first work list, cartons of printouts totaling more than 1,200 pages.

For direct identifications, on December 13 Gene Codes Forensics had delivered MFISys, which immediately replaced World Trade Center CODIS as our prime software tool for making direct identifications. The state police continued to store the STR data in the World Trade Center CODIS. Before the end of December, my group was making both direct and indirect (kinship) identifications. This system would remain intact for several months.

I had also set in motion my Phase III testing, although that's not how I referred to it at the time. John Butler was validating the Big

Mini. Celera Genomics was establishing a forensic mtDNA sequencing laboratory, and Orchid Cellmark in Dallas was revamping its SNP parentage test so that I could use it on DMs having fewer than 100 base pairs of DNA. I thought the prognosis for future identifications looked bright.

One of the most satisfying aspects of the World Trade Center effort was working with professionals much more intelligent than I. Mostly, their expertise differed from mine, which always guaranteed fertile and stimulating discussions. Mandy was one of these people.

From within this vortex of analytical activity, she recognized a critical need to define our work more carefully, suggesting emphatically to Howard Cash that Gene Codes Forensics create work lists from within MFISys, lists of potential identifications that we could confirm, place on hold for more data, or discard as a nonidentification. She correctly believed this would help to focus the work and streamline it by eliminating much of the redundancy. She was correct, of course.

Work lists did eventually come. The first came from Charles Brenner in DNAView, which was eventually imported into MFISys. Benoit Leclair created lists in MDKAP, and Steve Sherry, who was on the KADAP panel and worked for the National Center for Biological Informatics, created another. Each of these created different work lists. Mostly, the kinship work lists were similar, but there were enough differences that each found identifications the others missed.

Then Mandy went after the contract laboratories. Although each contract laboratory had a superb reputation and had passed mandatory inspections, Mandy thought we should have written procedures from each detailing their guidelines for accepting data. She was correct, of course.

Although we had checks and balances in place to review the data as we received it, obtaining written procedures with respect to what each laboratory considered "good" data had slipped through the cracks in the initial chaotic months.

Mandy extended her quality attack to the changing face of software iterations. She, Dr. Elizabeth Pugh, who was a part of the National Institutes of Health Human Genome Project at Johns Hopkins University, Steve Niezgoda, and Steve Sherry focused on new versions of the software.

Software was as important to the success of the project as the DNA testing, an essential part of the overall identification process. All of the DNA-matching software we were using, both kinship and direct, was being written on the fly, and we were receiving new versions weekly. Although those writing the code were competent software engineers, it is well documented that new versions of even commercial-grade software have bugs—anyone who upgrades to a new version of Windows is well aware of the pitfalls of upgrades.

We learned this lesson the hard way when new versions of DNAView gave different kinship statistics than prior versions. Elizabeth, Steve Sherry, Steve Niezgoda, and Mandy were concerned enough that they worked out standardized procedures to ensure that each new version of the software passed a test designed to ensure consistency from version to version. With the exception of MFISys, we had a rule: no one used new software until Steve Niezgoda blessed it.

In early April 2002, Steve and I began talking about another critical issue: missing samples. This first came to my attention while working on kinship identifications in the early mornings. For example, while working from either a DNAView or MDKAP work list, I would fail to find a DM in MFISys, although it should have been there. After finding a number of these inconsistencies, I mentioned it to Steve and Mandy.

As an error-checking exercise, each time we received data from the vendors, called a data dump, Steve checked the STR data in CODIS and then compared it with the data in MFISys. The total number of STR profiles should have been identical because MFISys imported the data directly from the WTC CODIS server in Albany. They were not, and it posed a problem.

Steve viewed the problem quantitatively. He e-mailed the following statistics to Mitch Holland at Bode: MFIsys had 5,261 DMs with full or partial DNA profiles and 1,154 DMs with no profiles for a total of 6,415 DMs. After comparing the Bode DM having the highest DM number in CODIS, he speculated that we had an apparent discrepancy of 8,189 DMs. At the end of the e-mail, Steve wrote, "So the question is, where are all the other samples?!?!"

Missing more than 8,000 DMs was a sickeningly disturbing problem. The few isolated missing samples I had noticed while doing kinship analyses had suddenly ballooned. How could we lose track of over 8,000 DMs? Steve thought the gaps resulted from the network and the BEAST not tracking DMs properly. I prayed this was correct. The effect on the families was something I preferred not to dwell on.

Tracking the source of the problem was challenging. We had no way to monitor the comings and goings of samples and data. The sixth-floor disaster team would send samples out the door using one tracking system, and data would come back on a separate data stream. Neither "talked" to the other. The STR typing data magically ended up in CODIS and then in MFISys. I had no way to correlate numbers of samples with STR data. Once I received the data, I had no way to check when the DNA extracts returned to the lab unless I singled out a particular DM and then asked Lydia for the information, which I had to do for a few DMs. Doing this manually for thousands would have been impossible.

DMs or family samples left the OCME or the state police respectively and went to a contract laboratory. The contract laboratory ran the STR profiles and then sent the data to the state police. What seemed like a simple process actually was not. Had we lost DMs, the data, or both? Like Steve, I believed we had a flaw in our counting system that we had to identify and then fix. A worst-case scenario meant we'd have to resample thousands of DMs and then reextract them.

Mitch's reply to Steve's e-mail was reassuring and provided part of the answer. He believed we would always have discrepancies. There would always be data outside of CODIS in the review process at the New York State Police or in transit from Bode or the OCME. He also suggested there would always be a DM count discrepancy because

Bode was continually pulling DMs out of the queue for reanalysis. Mitch's logic sounded reasonable and reassuring. But 8,189?

By April 30, Steve was still searching for the "missing" samples. Chris Cave at Bode told him the bone DMs giving low STR profiles or zero STR profiles data had never been sent to the New York State Police because of an ongoing software retooling project at Bode. Had we found the problem?

Steve set up a phone conference with the state police and Bode. Each laboratory counted all the DMs not tallied yet in CODIS, and we added up the numbers. Like magic, the total nearly equaled the number of missing DMs—all but six. Thank God.

Independently, Mandy got into the missing-sample fray. She had also expressed concern with what appeared to be a separate discrepancy. Actually, the problem really was a nonproblem because we had deliberately withheld approximately 300 DMs from CODIS due to extraction blank problems, which occurred when samples that were controls and should have been negative actually had data. Typically, Mandy sank her teeth into the problem and stirred the pot for a couple of days. Lydia eventually straightened out what, in the end, turned out to be a paper problem.

Extensive commingling had become a problem. We were receiving firefighters' remains with extra parts when remains came into the morgue in bunker gear. During the autopsy, the ME often found, for instance, two right femurs, which was impossible. On April 5, 2002, Mark Flomenbaum sent an e-mail to the medical examiners reminding them that remains having unattached pieces should be considered separate cases, even if found inside one article of clothing such as the New York City Fire Department bunker gear. If remains had several pieces that were not logically attached, that is, connected by tissue, they were to be separated and treated as separate DMs. When these situations occurred, Amy Mundorff resampled the duplicate remains and then sent them to the special-projects group in my lab for analysis.

22 THE END—BUT NOT FINISHED

May 31, 2002

Missing Identified: 853

DNA Identifications: 406

Pieces Reconciled: 2,250

We leaped into May 2002 full of anticipation that our string of new identifications would continue. It did, and it was wonderful.

After seven months of continuous work, the flurry of activity had amazingly increased. The resampling and reanalysis of remains requiring special attention continued unabated, the logistics and weekly family meetings continued, and revised alpha versions of DNAView continually plagued new identifications that had to be recalculated. A project I started in April to quality check the STR data ballooned, a hacker reputedly got into our MFISys server, and tracking DMs having zero-STR profiles remained a sticky issue. Shiya's RM-mapping project had located approximately 700 families with data problems. The mtDNA and SNP validation studies were delayed, the British decided to monitor our DNA effort, and the state police wanted out. The city wanted out, too. The mayor scheduled the closing ceremony at the World Trade Center site, which meant the city was calling it quits on the recovery effort.

In January 2002, I signed a kinship identification report identifying one of the World Trade Center missing persons. Or I thought I had. I sent the paperwork through Mike Hennessey's continually evolving admin review process. We reported the DNA identification to the medicolegal investigators, and they notified the New York City Police Department, which contacted the family. The family claimed the remains. Job well done, I thought. I did not know then that the person I thought I had identified had a brother who also perished on September 11.

Full siblings of the same sex (not identical twins) usually have different STR profiles, each of which fits the genetic mold of their family. However, without a direct-reference STR profile such as a toothbrush, it is impossible to know which brother had been identified. In this instance, I had identified a brother and had assigned a name to the DM. After learning about the other brother, I had a 50–50 chance I had been correct. Which brother had I sent home to his family? I did not know.

That there were two brothers and that both were missing was information I needed, information that should have been in the family collection records in Albany. But it wasn't. Even Albany did not realize both brothers were missing because the personal effects from both of them had been mixed together into the same evidence collection bag by the New York City Police Department at the Family Assistance Center. To the New York State Police, there was only one missing son in the family.

In March we identified the other brother using kinship analysis. It had to be a brother because the remains had a different STR profile from the brother I had identified in January. However, like the first identification, its STR profile fit snugly into the family's genetic structure. We had the proper family, of that we were certain, but we might have had a naming error. I hoped this would not mean another traumatic visit to a family. We had to solve the problem, if possible. Knowing we had the correct family offered some solace and knowing we had found both brothers offered hope.

Peter Wistort pulled the personal effects from both brothers and ran the DNA profiles on six additional personal effects, four of which gave complete STR profiles. According to Peter's records, a razor, a toothbrush, and a hairbrush had been attributed to one of the brothers. The DNA typing gave interesting results. The razor and the hairbrush had the same STR profile, but the toothbrush was different. Its STR profile matched the toothbrush that had been submitted for the other brother. In May, Peter wrote saying that he wasn't sure which profile belonged to which brother. This left me with no clear way to sort out the naming problem.

We kept digging into the records for any clue that might help, a process that took from March until July before we had the answer. Mike Hennessey found out that one of the two brothers had an electric razor. The electric razor's STR profile matched the remains we had returned to the family in January. Most important, we had given those remains the correct name. It was dumb luck, but I gladly accepted it.

We stored all of our important intake or chain-of-custody data electronically in files in a laboratory information system called the BEAST. Actually, we had two BEASTs. The one located at the OCME in my laboratory contained information relating to the DMs received from the World Trade Center site and the Fresh Kills landfill. It also tracked where we stored them in the laboratory and where we sent them for analysis. Lydia's sixth-floor disaster team maintained this system. The second BEAST resided in Albany and contained the family information collected by the NYPD at the Family Assistance Centers. There was no logical electronic connection between the two BEASTs, so the systems did not "talk" to each other. This created a nightmarish communication problem when we needed both data sets to make identifications.

At Steve's July 2002 logistics meetings Tom Brondolo, the OCME deputy commissioner who manages personnel, IT, and procurement, announced his decision to sunset—stop using—the BEAST and replace it with an in-house system he had been developing with a company called CCR. Called the Integrated Management System or simply the Integrated System, this system was to supplant the BEAST. Tom reasoned that switching systems would save the city the expense of maintaining the BEAST. He planned to make this happen in September 2002.

I couldn't believe what I was hearing. Steve and I glanced at each other. We were thinking the same thing: How would we work without the BEAST? This was an incredible revelation, one without warning, and I had to work hard to keep my annoyance hidden. I asked Tom, "How long before the Integrated System is ready?"

Tom and Raju Venkataram, the director of the OCME IT department, exchanged what appeared to be an uncomfortable glance. "Three weeks," Raju said nervously.

I thought, Okay, three weeks, I can deal with that. Actually, I really did not have a choice, but three weeks sounded reasonable, so I was willing to give them a chance to succeed.

The philosophy behind the Integrated System made sense. Theoretically, the system could pull in multiple databases simultaneously, which if they were updated regularly, meant we would have more and varied information on our desktops. Shiya had been working with Tom and Raju and with CCR to create the system, so it was his expertise and experience that formed the basis of its functionality—tasks it could perform. The CCR software engineers (in residence at the OCME) under Raju's direction did the coding. Ideally, a completed Integrated System should have made the second-floor World Trade Center DNA identification unit's work more efficient.

Tom's plan was more ambitious, however. His idea was to move the Integrated System from a simple data interface to a fully functional LIMS system. Unfortunately, the Integrated System's databases were not updated frequently enough to be useful, which meant critical information was not always readily available. The Integrated System was meant to be used by anyone working on the World Trade Center project, not just the DNA laboratory. So developing a system in a short time that was all things to everyone using it was nearly impossible.

The CODIS and BEAST files eventually made it into the Integrated System. However, the data from MFISys, our most important DNA database, never made it into the system. This meant that the Integrated System never completely addressed the second-floor World Trade Center DNA identification group's needs. Also, as mtDNA and SNP data became available, the Integrated System couldn't handle them either. So the three most important DNA databases never became a part of the Integrated System.

Equally troublesome, at first, was that the Integrated System would not permit ad hoc searches. So when I or anyone in Elaine's second-floor unit needed a special search, we had to ask Raju to run the search for us, which he did willingly. Unfortunately, this took time, and we often needed the information much quicker. Eventually, Mike Hennessey was given the ability to run his own searches.

I needed the Integrated System operational in July 2002, the same month Tom announced his decision. The promised three weeks came and went. A month came and went. In fact, a completely functional Integrated System was not available until June 2003, a year late.

Whether the reasons for the delays were justifiable or not, I do not know, because I was not privy to the pressures on Tom or Raju. However, I thought the delay was inexcusable and grossly insensitive to the families. Frustrated by the delays, I ordered Lydia to continue using the BEAST.

Steve's logistics meeting in early May 2002 was disappointing.

Barry Duceman's group in Albany was the first to show that re-analyzing the DNA extracts from personal effects gave a high percentage of samples that previously had given poor or no STR results. They had taken DNA extracts returned from Myriad and reanalyzed them. Many of these yielded STR profiles good enough to make identifications. He wanted permission to reanalyze a large number of personal effects and had targeted 95 of the 170 batches to rework. This represented almost 9,000 samples, a huge unanticipated challenge for the state police. Unanticipated commitments, it seemed, had become the hallmark of the World Trade Center effort for all of us.

Barry originally thought he could complete the DNA typing of the 95 batches by the end of May 2002. However, since there was limited or no DNA extract remaining from many of the personal effects, someone would have to track down the original personal effects, reexamine them, reextract the DNA, run the STRs, and then load the data into the World Trade Center CODIS. He did not have the resources. Realizing this, he said, "We can't promise we'll be finished before the end of September—maybe October."

In essence, he was saying that the STR data from the personal effects would not be available to make identifications until sometime in the fall, which he knew would upset me because I had made it clear to the contract laboratories that I wanted to conclude the Phase II DNA work by the first anniversary. To do this, I needed the DNA data from the personal effects so that we could make new identifications.

It was a blow. He was extending the process, and I certainly did not want to wait until October or November. As it turned out, it really didn't matter because the bulk of the DNA work would not be completed until spring 2004, when we received the last batch of SNP data. I was sitting next to Steve when Barry made the announcement.

The take-home message for me was that the state police weren't willing to allocate more resources to the World Trade Center effort. The state police wanted out as soon as possible. Barry spelled it out: the extra effort would tie up analysts' time, analysts who were supposed to be working on criminal cases, which was, after all, the New York State Police mission. The World Trade Center work, however, was important and had to get done. Who would do it?

Bringing in another public forensic laboratory to analyze the 9,000 samples was illogical. Most public labs do not have the resources to integrate an additional 9,000 samples into their testing system, which meant I would need to enlist several laboratories. Private labs were a possibility, but I did not have a contract with another private lab that I felt could do the work reliably. Also, it would have been tough finding one quickly at such a late date. Bode's plate was full, as was Orchid's, and I was reluctant to add more to their burden.

I took a deep breath. "We'll do it," I said, trying to make my voice sound like it was no big deal. But it was. It was huge.

My lab had been steadily assuming an increasing World Trade Center burden. Our special-projects group had a burgeoning workload. We were reanalyzing tissue samples, almost 3,000 of them, much like Barry had proposed for the personal effects. Like him, I had an even larger casework burden and increasing pressure to turn out homicide and sexual-assault cases in a timely fashion.

As the discussion wore on, I realized that Barry was uncomfortable with the decision to pull the plug. He even apologized months later. Certainly this had not been his decision, but it was devastating and would affect the project and my laboratory. The state police had been anxious to help on September 11, going to great lengths to ensure they were included in the effort. They had asked for the responsibility for the family samples and had been a tremendous help during a tough time. But their promise to stick by us to the bitter end never materialized. My laboratory had to suck it up like it had been doing since September 11. We would do the work ourselves.

Mark Desire had managed the analysis of the family samples from the American Airlines Flight 587 crash. Now he had to assume the responsibility for the World Trade Center family sample reanalysis project.

The World Trade Center site officially closed on May 31, nearly four months shy of the first September 11 anniversary. Although the Staten Island landfill at Fresh Kills remained open, the closing ceremony at the World Trade Center site represented the city's official culmination of a heroic effort to recover the missing.

The mayor's office asked the city agencies involved in the rescue, recovery, and identification efforts to send representatives to the ceremony. I was chosen as one of five to represent the OCME. I felt proud to be a part of it. The entire world was going to witness the end of a difficult and trying process. With the exception of the families, most of the world would watch the ceremony on TV and believe it marked the end of the recovery and identification process. This chapter in their lives would close, and they would move on and focus on rebuilding their lives. It was a false end, though. The digging at the World Trade Center site had ended, but our work had not.

It turned out to be a hot, sunny day. Tom Brondolo, Shiya Ribowsky, and I stood on the ramp leading into the World Trade Center excavation site. We weren't sure what was expected of us, so we waited for more than an hour baking in the heat, chatting nervously.

When the ceremony began, I was transfixed by what happened. I can't remember the exact sequence of events, but at the end, each of the recovery-rescue workers marched out of the "pit" and passed us. When John Cartier, brother of James Cartier and a member of the family that started the family group Give Your Voice, passed me, tears sprung up uncontrollably. I remember saying something, I don't remember what. He acknowledged me but kept walking, his face stoic and sad.

After the parade of rescuers passed, it was our turn to march out. Not knowing where we were going, we followed the queue, passing Mayor Giuliani, Mayor Bloomberg, and Governor George Pataki onto West Street. We passed crowds of cheering, respectful, and grateful people who lined the streets from West Street north. Sweat oozed from my every pore, and it seemed like a journey that would never end. When we finally finished, I was emotionally drained and drenched.

I had to force back tears for most of the march. I tried hard to be strong, but as I studied the tear-streaked faces of people lining the streets, I noticed something that ripped at my heart. It was love. A city known for its toughness and rough exterior had fallen in love, with us. I still choke up when I remember it.

A thought had been filtering through my mind throughout the ceremony. The city and the nation remembered only the heroic efforts of the firefighters, the most publicized of those at the recovery-rescue effort. And the cheers were mostly for them. I certainly do not begrudge them that honor. They were heroes, though heroism had seemed to acquire new meaning after September 11. I could not help thinking that the nameless, faceless heroes who worked to identify the missing were never mentioned or acknowledged, except by those few who understood.

Still, it was a very special day, one I will never forget.

23 A POLICY CHANGE AND A FUNERAL

June 25, 2002

Missing Identified: 1,203

DNA Identifications: 495

Pieces Reconciled: 3,463

When the World Trade Center site officially closed, I expected more scrutiny of the DNA operations. Questions such as, "Why is DNA taking so long?" or "How many more will you identify?" had been on the media's collective mind, and I expected them to increase. The Fresh Kills landfill was still being operated, and I was hoping that activity would shield me. I had my doubts. Reporters now had only the OCME as an outlet for the most relevant World Trade Center statistic: how many had we identified?

The questions about SNPs had been filtering in, fueled, I believe, by Orchid's apparent need for publicity in the wake of its financial woes. It seemed that articles about Orchid's involvement with the World Trade Center work kept cropping up, which seemed premature to me because the company had not completed its validation experiments. I was concerned whether we would ever use SNPs. In contrast, the other vendors—Bode, Gene Codes Forensics, and Myriad—had been careful not to reach out to the media.

Orchid's financial situation had me worried. I had the nagging feeling that the company's ability to support the World Trade Center effort might go the same path as the state police. The key difference was that my laboratory did not have the expertise to do the SNP testing, so we would not be able to pick up the slack. I did speak to Bob Giles about it, and he assured me that his company was in it for the long run. He was true to his word and, thankfully, my fears were unfounded.

Also unfounded were my fears about the media focusing on the OCME. A few reporters maintained a keen interest, but the vast majority had moved on to other, more contemporary topics. Fine with me.

Throughout the World Trade Center effort, the OCME assumed the pragmatic position that because anyone working on the project is human, mistakes are expected. As Chuck Hirsch liked to say, "Nothing in my job description says I'm not human." As with any complex endeavor, it was inevitable. We made it our credo. However, we were also determined to learn from our mistakes. We established new policies so they could not happen again. Mark Flomenbaum's April 5, 2002, e-mail to the medical examiners requiring them to separate remains not logically attached was one such example. It stemmed from a case that hit me and others especially hard, so much so that it spawned a comprehensive anthropological reexamination of all remains before returning them to families.

It was mid-April and almost the end of the day. I was beat and looking for an excuse to leave. I had just about convinced myself that I had finished for the day when Amy Mundorff, our resident anthropologist, appeared at my office door. Her expression told me she had a problem. She came in and shut the door, something she rarely did, so I knew something was wrong. She immediately swore me to secrecy, saying she had to get something off her chest. I thought she was going to tell me about a fight she had with Shiya or one of the MEs about collecting evidence in the morgue. Sometimes she seemed at loggerheads with them. But her problem was not that simple.

She had just returned from examining the remains of someone who had worked in 2 World Trade Center. DNA had identified him by matching the profile of one of the remains to DNA taken from a razor. Slam dunk, I thought. The look on her face said something else.

"Don't tell me we fucked up the identification!" I said.

"No," she said.

Thankfully, it was another problem, the first of its kind.

After being notified, the family wanted to know what was left of their loved one; a reasonable and common enough request. It is important to understand that the remains were not the property of the City of New York, and a family had the right to any we had identified. Amy routinely examined the remains at Memorial Park before turning them over to a family, so she was the last stop between getting it right and sending remains home. I often wondered whether anyone less motivated, concerned, or conscientious would have been as diligent.

In this instance, there was a torso, upper and lower, and both parts had been described by the ME who did the autopsy. Packaged with the torso, the ME found a pair of right hands, which she correctly separated, giving each a different DM number. It had been, from the start, a typical case of commingling. Obviously, two people had died together. Although the ME assigned the upper and lower torsos a single DM number, she collected muscle from each and submitted both specimens to the DNA lab, standard operating procedure so far.

Amy was concerned that the upper and lower torsos might be from two different people. If that were true, and if we did not separate them, a family would receive someone else's remains, perhaps the only remains of that person recovered, and the second family might never receive their loved one.

I listened carefully and thought it should be simple enough to find out whether the torsos came from one or two people. She had not mentioned DNA, so I assumed she had not checked to see whether the upper and lower torsos had the same STR profile. The problem emerged when she started searching out the DNA profiles of the two torsos. I had to check the DNA for myself and naïvely thought it was a matter of checking MFISys to sort out the problem. I got into the MFISys database and found that there were actually three matching pieces, all with full DNA profiles, more than statistically sufficient to make the identification. Simply examining the DNA profiles did not send up a red flag. The next step was to check the OCME BEAST to see what DMs had been received into the laboratory.

Amy and I went into the lab, where I was surprised to find Elaine Mar standing at the BEAST workstation working on the same problem. She had already learned that we had received two samples, one from each torso. The problem was that MFISys had a single STR profile for only one of the torsos. Now I was concerned. Then Chuck Hirsch strode into the lab. Another surprise. We discussed the situation briefly, and he decided to have everyone working on the case meet in his office.

When we were there, Chuck explained why he thought both torsos should be released to the family. He reminded us that the New York City Fire Department's well-intentioned though innovative World Trade Center site meddling—putting loose remains into bunker gear—had jaded us unnecessarily, which he thought might be clouding our better judgment. He also reminded us that our job was to make identifications to a reasonable degree of scientific certainty. No one expected us to go beyond that level, a standard he thought we might be applying in this case. He was correct, of course; there are no absolute certainties in the mass-fatality identification business, just probabilities.

Amy stood her ground. She reminded us that the medical examiner who conducted the autopsy, an extremely competent observer, had described the torso as "upper and lower torso parts," implying the torsos were separated entities, and had purposely collected samples from both. Not lost on the medical examiner was the unnerving fact that two right hands had also been submitted with the torsos, which meant that, minimally, two people's remains had been commingled either when the buildings fell or during the recovery. Amy reasoned further that, although the medical examiner had given both torsos the same DM number, something about the case had warranted collecting a DNA specimen from each torso. Either that or she was simply being extremely careful because of the two right hands. Either way, Amy was uneasy giving both torsos to the family without additional investigation.

I shared her concern and added that the laboratory should have DNA extracts in the freezer and that we could begin testing the extracts that day with DNA results the next morning. I asked Chuck to wait until then before calling the family. He agreed.

I returned to the lab and asked Lydia to have someone reanalyze the extracts from both torsos. Then we discovered another problem. When she went to locate them, she learned that we had only one of the two extracts. The other was missing! According to the BEAST both DMs should have been there. I was stunned. How could we have lost one of the extracts?

I spoke to Zoran Budimlija, a free-spirited pathologist who was also special projects supervisor, and asked him to go with Amy to Memorial Park and resample both torsos. Lydia found the original DMs from both torsos in the freezer, the ones the medical examiner originally collected. Thank God we had them. The disaster team extracted the DNA from the original samples sent to the lab by the medical examiner. Zoran took the newly collected samples from Amy and extracted them. He amplified the extracts, and Chris Kamnik read the results the next morning. At 10:00 A.M., Zoran gave me the bottom line.

The STR profiles did not match. The torsos were from different people.

The lower torso belonged to the family who had requested the information, and the upper torso belonged to someone we had yet to meet. This hit me hard. I went to the first-floor conference room to tell Shiya. As I entered the room, all talking ceased. The medicolegal investigators turned toward me, and as I conveyed what we had found, they stared at me for a moment and then started to clap. I was stunned. When I called Chuck and gave him the news, I thought I heard him exhale. I still choke up when I think of a family never receiving that upper torso. We identified the other torso months later.

Although Craig Venter left Celera Genomics in January 2002, I didn't hear about it until February, and my heart sank. Since he had been the vehicle for Celera being involved in the World Trade Center work, I immediately had visions of the mtDNA effort crashing down. The entire mitochondrial effort would become an expensive exercise, not to mention possibly dashing the hopes of families who had yet to receive the remains of their loved ones. The thought haunted me. I never expected mtDNA sequencing would be a magic wand that would produce new identifications, but I did expect it would point us in the direction of several new ones once we neared the end of the project.

Thinking back to the exciting conversation I had had with Craig on September 12, 2001, I now had only one thought: had Craig's excitement and Celera's promise duped me? His and Celera's reputation had lured me, no question. Once again I had gotten myself into a mess, one I thought had redefined the paradigm of how to use mtDNA in mass-fatality investigations. Nine months later, I was still waiting for the Celera promise, and this news left me wondering whether the company would deliver.

Except for an oral commitment to the World Trade Center families, Celera could legally walk away from the project because the City of New York had not finalized its contract. On top of that, Celera's new president, Cathy Ordonez, had asked for a face-to-face conference. I was expecting the worst. From the very first Kinship and Data Analysis Panel meeting, the mtDNA effort had become a monumental project and was, at best, complicated.

Celera Genomics is part of the Applera umbrella, which includes the biotechnology company Applied Biosystems. When I gave Celera the go-ahead in September 2001, Applied Biosystems appointed Rhonda Roby the project manager and transferred her from Foster City, California (Applied Biosystems's headquarters), to Celera at

Rockville, Maryland. Having once been a forensic DNA scientist experienced in mtDNA sequencing when she worked at the Armed Forces DNA Identification Lab, Rhonda had been a logical candidate to head Celera's World Trade Center mtDNA effort. Rhonda's Celera group dubbed the project "Soaring Eagles."

Rhonda dove into the project with the enthusiasm of a young kid. In hindsight, she probably had the company and its scientists jump through more hoops than necessary, but these efforts only strengthened Celera's credibility, in my opinion. Under her direction, the company constructed, from scratch and at substantial cost, a true forensic mitotyping laboratory. She insisted that the Celera scientists meet the federal DNA Advisory Board qualifications for forensic DNA scientists, to the extent that she had them testify in mock trials—not that anyone actually expected they would ever testify.

Not unexpectedly but certainly frustrating from my viewpoint, Soaring Eagles had a slow start. Although many members of the KADAP had a healthy skepticism about Celera's ability to do the work, the scientists in the company were enthusiastic. Rhonda's early projections had the mtDNA work beginning by November 2001, which left Howard Baum scratching his head. Even I, the most impatient person in the world, realized this was an enthusiast's dream. Celera had a long row to hoe. The mtDNA subcommittee of the KADAP skeptically watched as Celera went through the motions to validate its stake in the World Trade Center work.

Howard Baum oversaw the mito effort, and the KADAP mitochondrial subcommittee demanded that Celera take a blind proficiency test. This is a laboratory exercise administered to test a laboratory's ability to obtain reliable results under specified conditions. For the World Trade Center work, this exercise consisted of compromised tissue. Only Howard Baum at the OCME knew the correct answers to the test. Bode and Celera took the tests, and Howard compared their results. Howard sent Celera and Bode seventy-five samples from the American Airlines Flight 587 disaster.

The results were blind to both companies, which meant they did not know the origin of the samples. We had done extensive STR testing on the samples, so we knew which samples belonged together. Howard had the Bode Technology Group take the test because I wanted Bode to be a backup in those situations where Celera had problems or if we needed to confirm a Celera mitotype.

Howard compared the results and found no mitotyping discrepancies between the two laboratories. On June 18, 2002, Dr. Anne Walsh of the NYS Department of Health gave Celera the go-ahead to begin mtDNA testing. It was a grand moment, and not too far off my original target date to begin mtDNA testing. It also officially marked the beginning of Phase III testing and our employment of alternate DNA technologies such as miniplexes and SNPs.

However, after Craig Venter left Celera, I noticed a shift in the company's dedication to Soaring Eagles. After a couple of meetings with corporate officers, both from Celera and Applied Biosystems, I felt strongly that they wanted out at the first face-saving opportunity. No one explicitly said it like that, but their intent was clear to me.

The first of the meetings took place in March. I met with Cathy Ordonez, Celera's president; Ugo DeBlasi, Celera's chief financial officer; and Rhonda. Cathy wanted two things: the total number of World Trade Center and personal effect samples they would receive from the OCME and a time line when they would have all the samples in-house.

The second meeting occurred months later and included Applied Biosystems officials. Rhonda was conspicuously absent. Surprisingly, by this time, Applied Biosystems had effectively removed her from the project's daily management. In my opinion, the company was trying to limit its financial exposure by defining the extent of the mtDNA testing. They never asked out of Craig Venter's original commitment, but they clearly sought to define and limit their tasks.

Paradoxically, I thought Celera was doing the right thing. They certainly had a right to pursue their business as they saw fit and, by defining and assessing their risk, they were being responsible to their shareholders.

I am not privy to Applied Biosystems's corporate strategies, nor should I be, but what bothered me most was when they transferred Rhonda back to Foster City, ripping her physically from the Soaring Eagles management. Her replacement, Dr. Mark Adams, a brilliant computer scientist and a Celera vice president, certainly competent in his field, is neither a forensic scientist nor an experienced forensic mtDNA sequencing expert. The end result was that Applied Biosystems had effectively left me naked and the World Trade Center mtDNA effort potentially exposed to error. To make the situation worse, Rhonda was forced to work on the World Trade Center project on her own time. Phone calls were made after hours and e-mails came from her home computer.

With Celera pushing to wind down, I feared I no longer had an mtDNA-sequencing laboratory, a thought that haunted me until I realized that my plan had always included a backup, Bode. My plan was to determine as many family and personal effects mitotypes as possible. With this data in MFISys, we could match these mitotypes with mitotypes from DMs, which I hoped would point us in the direction of an appropriate family.

There were other ways to utilize mtDNA to make or help make identifications. Because of the large number of partial STR profiles we obtained, I expected many of the potential kinship or direct matches would not meet the KADAP statistical barrier using STRs or SNPs alone. But adding a mitotype might boost the statistics sufficiently to make an identification. For example, if a kinship identification had a matching statistic that was close, a mitotype that matched a relative gave us confidence that we had the correct family. Also, if a mitotype matched a personal effect where the STR data did not make the KADAP minimum, the mitotype bolstered the statistics. Noelle Umback, an OCME criminalist supervising scientist, used this approach to make several identifications.

I also thought we could use mtDNA to narrow the search for identifications. From MFISys we could obtain a list of families having the same mitotype (approximately 7 percent of Caucasians have the same mitotype). This approach effectively trimmed the potential universe of families we had to search. Armed with this information, we could use STRs or SNPs to further narrow the list of candidate families. Deciding which family to target required additional work.

When a mitotype was critical to making an identification, my original plan was to ask Bode to resequence the DM. If the Celera and Bode mitotypes matched, I thought we could be confident that the mitotype was correct. If I needed to resequence any of the DMs because the Celera typing was incomplete, I thought Bode could do that as well. So even though Celera seemed to want out of the WTC work, I expected the company would produce thousands of mitotypes that we could search against, and if we needed additional help, I planned to turn to Bode. Essentially, my mtDNA plan remained intact. Celera finally delivered the last of the World Trade Center mtDNA data in January 2004. By then, I had hired Rhonda as an OCME consultant because she had resigned from Applied Biosystems.

Never had I experienced such an avalanche of emotion as I did at James Cartier's funeral. Fran came into the city on Friday morning, June 20, so we could attend his funeral the next day. By happenstance, Lorraine Kelly had arranged an OCME evening dinner cruise on the East River, which gave us a well-deserved chance to relax and socialize for a few hours. We had been working at a grueling pace, and it was the first time since September 11 we had had a chance to unwind.

I had mentioned the Cartiers to Fran several times, so she knew the family had a special relationship with several of us at the OCME. This would be the first time she would meet them. On Friday afternoon, Fran, Tom Brondolo, and I took the OCME van to the funeral home in Queens for James's viewing.

It is important to point out how working in a continuously emotionally charged environment had affected me. Constant exposure, for twelve or fourteen hours a day, left me drained. After work, I found it next to impossible to rehash the day's activities. I often wanted to be alone, go to bed, watch something meaningless on TV, or chug a couple of drinks just to ease the tension. Mostly, I wanted to be alone, and I had very little to say.

When Fran would ask, "How'd your day go?" I might have said something like, "The Cartiers came to Memorial Park to view their brother's remains," without elaborating or explaining. I simply had no desire to relive it.

Typically, Fran would ask, "Are you all right?"

"Yeah," I'd lie, still roiling inside. I usually tried to change the subject and get her to talk about her day so that my mind could curl up into an emotional ball, which effectively put the kibosh on a meaningful conversation. Sometimes I related something that happened at a family meeting. Mostly, though, these were disjointed conversations that taken out of context were hard for anyone to weave into anything coherent. It wasn't until James's funeral that Fran could sew it together, and it was not until she met the Cartier family that she truly understood. Witnessing the affection between the OCME staff and the family drove home how special and close this relationship had become, one that transcended the official OCME function of identifying James.

The viewing room at the funeral home held chairs for at least one hundred people. I scanned the room, looking for the Cartier family. James's parents sat in front facing the closed casket, which was covered with an American flag. His brothers Patrick and John were greeting people at the door. His sister Michele stood closest, and I immediately went to her. We hugged and then I introduced Fran. Next I saw Michael, Marie, Patrick, and John, in that order. By the time we'd made it to James's father and I introduced Fran, I was a wreck.

We stayed long enough to pay our respects. When we were ready to leave, we spent time with James's sister Marie, who is a delightful and thoughtful young woman. She entertained us, lightening the tension a bit by sharing her efforts to secure the Jacob Javits Center for the families' One Day of Remembrance gathering they were planning. We returned to the OCME, where I met with Howard Cash for an hour. The next morning we drove to Our Lady of Fatima's Church in Queens for James's funeral.

Arriving early, I parked the car near the church and asked one of the IBEW Motorcycle Club members if we were parked in the right place. The IBEW is the International Brotherhood of Electrical Workers Local 103. This was James's union and his motorcycle club. He and his brother were proud members. It was a warm, sunny day, so being outside was nice, and I had no desire to be the first inside the church. Soon I heard a loud rumble. I turned in time to see bike after bike roar down 25th Street in a military-like sequence. Each biker angled his bike into the sidewalk and then they hung out, talking among themselves.

I watched Jack Lynch and his wife Cathleen, who lost their fire-fighter son Michael, park their SUV across the street. I first met Jack when we were discussing his son's remains, which had been found in bunker gear. There were multiple duplicate fragments, the hallmark of commingling. We explained to Jack that additional DNA testing would be necessary in order to identify Michael's remains, which meant that returning Michael's remains to him would take time. The special-projects group did the work.

While Jack and Cathleen waited for traffic to clear before crossing the road to the church, an OCME truck stopped. Katie Sullivan and Howard Cash got out. I was a little surprised to see Howard, but that was only a fleeting thought. He seemed to turn up everywhere, a fact that was reinforced over time. They walked over to us, and we stood in a small group for several minutes.

Finally, a hearse stopped in front of the church, so we went inside and sat in the seventh row from the front, close to the Cartier family. Bill Doyle, a Staten Island family representative who lost his son at the World Trade Center and was also a member of Give Your Voice— the family group started by the Cartiers—and his wife sat in front of us. Minutes later, Richie Scherer, Mayor Giuliani's director of the Office of Emergency Management on September 11, entered from a side door. I went to him. We shook hands, chatted briefly, and then went to the back of the church to greet Jennie, Marie, and Michele. Richie sat with us.

Minutes later the wailing sound of bagpipes filled the air. A chill coursed through me as I turned toward the back of the church. The Cartiers and their spouses were carrying James's casket solemnly into the church. They stopped midway down the aisle and waited until the priest gave a blessing. Then they moved the casket a short distance and set it down just at the end of the pews in front of the altar.

I glanced at Fran. Her eyes were red. Katie already had an emotionally spent look, and the service had not even started. I had to work hard to keep my emotions in check. During the service, Patrick mentioned our work at the OCME. Richie slapped my leg, and I started to cry. When Jennie read her father's poem "Tell the Nation," it ripped at my heart. Then Michael ended the tribute to his brother with "Happy birthday, James."

The processional to the cemetery was a different story. It seemed more like a car chase in an action film than a funeral motorcade. The motorcycles rode two abreast behind the hearse and the Cartier family cars. The rest of us had to keep up and fend for ourselves. The motorcyclists and/or the New York City Police Department blocked intersections so the funeral motorcade could remain intact, but once the motorcycles passed, they left their posts and allowed the traffic to flow, which left us to duke it out with merging and crossing traffic. Several of the intersections quickly turned into a battle of nerves and determination. I had no idea how to get to the cemetery, so I had to keep up or get lost. Even asking directions would be futile since I did not know the cemetery's name. But we got there.

We stood around the grave site and waited. Soon, the bagpipers began playing and there was a short ceremony. The sun was shining and it was warm. I felt like I belonged.

24 THE FIRST ANNIVERSARY

September 16, 2002
Missing Identified: 1,469
DNA Identifications: 673

The first anniversary of the September 11 attacks arrived at about the same time as the second-floor World Trade Center DNA identification unit turned out the 670th DNA identification. The KADAP had met on the tenth, scheduled so that panel members could attend the ceremony at the World Trade Center site. The year had flown by, it seemed, and I marveled at how much we had accomplished. I wish we could have done more, faster. I was apprehensive about attending. The emotional memories of the closing ceremony in May still haunted me, and I suspected this might be more difficult.

I met Tom Brondolo and Raju Venkataram, the OCME MIS director, at the OCME at about 6:00 A.M., and an OCME driver took us downtown to the corner of West and Albany Streets across from the World Trade Center site. We checked in with attendants who were seated inside a series of small colored tents that lined Albany Street. Hundreds of people were milling around wondering what to do. We received identification tags and were instructed to hang them around our necks. Officially, I was one of five OCME representatives slated to be the World Trade Center Honor Guard for the ceremony. I had no idea what that meant or what was expected of us.

Then some guy yelled, "Everyone with A on their ID, line up over here!"

He directed us to queue up according to our identification tags. Mine was labeled Ramp A, so I lined up with others having the same tag. There were five different tags, A to E, and a separate line formed for each. There might have been at least one hundred people in each line. Once the lines were in place, a security guard escorted us, in tandem, into the World Trade Center site, down the entrance ramp into the "pit"—the hole remaining after the rubble from the World Trade Center buildings had been removed. It is surrounded by concrete walls, or slurry walls, that were the foundation of the World Trade Center site and that keep the Hudson River from flooding the area. These walls form what is also known as the "bathtub." We were ushered into a large tent where they instructed us to wait until we were called.

Inside the tent were rows of folding chairs. Danish, coffee, milk, and fruit juices were served on a long table along the north side. TVs tuned to news channels were suspended from the tent posts on the opposite side. Tom and I sat and waited. Nothing was happening, and I was immediately restless. It was also sweltering inside the tent, which only exacerbated my uneasiness. I went outside where it was cooler. I met a female Coast Guard sailor who was having a cigarette. We chatted a bit, and I went back inside the tent, where I downed a sweet Danish along with a cup of coffee.

After about an hour, someone yelled, "Group A! Line up outside the tent!"

Like good soldiers, we did exactly that and then stood in the baking sun for what seemed like a long time, but which was probably only about fifteen minutes. Someone handed each of us a number—mine was 90—and told us that we had to line up in this precise order each time they called our group.

After more milling about, they marched us into the middle of the pit to a large circle surrounding a smaller wooden circular structure. I believe the wooden structure was either physically at the entrance to the World Trade Center or was symbolic of it. I did not know why it was there, but I would soon.

They instructed us to stand on green crosses painted in the dirt and told us that this was the exact spot where we were to stand each time we entered the pit. I'd guess we were ten to twenty yards from the wooden structure. I did not realize this was simply a dress rehearsal. After showing us how to march into the pit and where we were to stand, they marched us back to the tent and instructed us to wait.

About an hour later, someone yelled, "Group A!"

This time it was for real.

My stomach tightened. Once again, we formed our line outside the tent and waited as the guides ensured we were in the proper queue. After a few minutes, we marched to the center of the World Trade Center site and stood on our green crosses. I looked toward the ramp and noticed that our circle of honor guard opened at the base, which led into the pit. Nothing happened for a long time. Then, as if on cue, the wind picked up. Although it was a hot day, there was a constant, sometimes blustery breeze kicking up the dust in the pit and swirling it around, sometimes high into the air.

Groups of people started walking slowly down the ramp. There were only a few at first, but they were quickly followed by a continuous stream of people. At first, I wasn't sure who they were. They certainly did not look like city dignitaries; they were dressed too casually. Then it dawned on me. They were the next of kin, relatives, and friends of those who had died.

They carried roses, bouquets, funeral sprays, photos, and other memorabilia. Timidly, it seemed, they stepped from the ramp onto the dirt, entered the circled area surrounded by the honor guard, and headed toward the wooden structure. Now I understood.

We, the honor guard, were to be a human barrier that marked the boundaries beyond which the family members were not supposed to venture. City officials had decided, for insurance purposes, I suppose, that family members should not be wandering around the World

Trade Center site. As time went on, however, the families went where they wanted. Who was I to stop a grieving family member from exploring the place where his/her loved one had died?

What happened next amazed me, and it is something I still think about.

This seemingly unending stream of families filed into the circular area surrounded by the honor guard. Most went directly into the open circular area bordered by the wooden structure and strolled leisurely around the shrine, examining what others coming before them had left. Most stopped at a photo they recognized for several moments. Sometimes they cried, sometimes they embraced, and sometimes I could hear hushed conversation among them. Many did not even speak.

They tucked flowers into the openings that had been cut along the top of the wooden shrine and leaned floral bouquets, posters, and photos against it. Then after leaving a memento, they stood back and allowed their emotions to flow. Many cried openly. Others simply hung their heads, shaking them slowly.

Their grief was exhausting, and while I tried to remain detached and not watch, it was impossible. At first, I wiped tears from my eyes before they rolled down my cheeks, then I did not bother.

In short order, the families transformed the wooden shrine into an amazing, colorful display of affection, love, and grief. Posters and photos lay against it on the ground. I could not see an empty space for another photo or flower. The magic of the World Trade Center families had converted a simple wooden structure into a blooming symbol of love. Though the analogy might not be appropriate, I couldn't help comparing in a small way this simple structure with the simple carpenter Jesus, whose love transformed an entire civilization.

After paying their respects, the families left the circle inside the shrine and walked around the area between the honor guard and the shrine. Many formed small family prayer groups. Others constructed miniature shrines in the dirt using rocks from the pit to build small mounds into which they inserted a single rose, a bouquet, a flag. Many stuck photos of their loved ones into the dirt. Firefighters' families were distinctive. They wore purple orchid leis around their necks. One woman knelt beside her small shrine, laid her purple lei on the ground, surrounding the rose she had stuck in the dirt. She stared at it for several minutes, then lovingly removed petals from the lei and from the rose and laid them into what I suppose was a diary to preserve them. She stood, photographed the shrine, then walked away.

A few yards away from her, a young man and a woman—I guessed from their appearance that she was his mother—knelt next to a small shrine composed of several roses and a photo of a young man. I had trouble discerning the details. They remained there for some time, holding each other and looking down. After a while, the mother walked away while the young man remained behind looking down at the shrine and the photo. Then he set his jaw, clenched his fist, and thumped it hard against his chest.

Many family members recognized me and made it a point to talk. Our conversations were brief, but they made me feel so very special. These people are the salt of the earth, the best in the world. They have all been so gracious to me and to my staff and so grateful for the work we are doing for them.

Then it was God's turn.

The wind, which had been gusty all afternoon, suddenly turned fierce. It whipped through the pit with a fury that caught everyone's attention. Dirt swirled around me like an angry ghost, lashing at my face and stinging my eyes. Then, as if someone had yanked it out of the pit, the swirling maelstrom soared skyward as if being pulled to heaven by a powerful force. It was eerie. Many of us remarked that it reminded us of the huge dust cloud that had formed when the Twin Towers fell. It was both frightening and breathtaking, a powerful moment that we all felt: God had released the spirits. When it was finally over, I was filthy from the dirt beating against my face and clothes. Yet I felt cleansed and calm. I believe those unfortunate people who died at that spot had finally found peace. That they were resting in a better place.

After I retired, Fran and I returned to the WTC site with my sister Kathi and her son Lee and his girlfriend, Sam, during the Fourth of July weekend, 2005. As I explained how the wind had grabbed the dust in the pit and pulled it skyward, the same emotion hit me again, and I had to take a couple of quick breaths in order to finish explaining what had happened.

25 2003: THE FIRST SIX MONTHS

June 25, 2003

Missing Identified: 1,508

DNA Identifications: 769

Total Pieces Reconciled: 6,588

DNA Direct Matches: 2,672

DNA Kinship Identifications: 1,643

DNA Direct and Kinship Identifications: 1,724

DNA Identifications Not Specified: 531

January 2003 started much like December ended; Elaine's second-floor group continued piecing together identifications, accumulating inestimable hours enduring incalculable emotional stress. Lydia's sixth-floor disaster team remained completely immersed in another massive tissue reextraction project, with the DNA extracts slated to go to Orchid Biosciences in Dallas for SNP testing.

People outside the OCME often asked, "How are you doing?"

My canned reply was, "We're still working on the World Trade Center." At other times, I'd say, "We're still knee-deep in the World Trade Center effort." Their response was almost predictable. There would be a prolonged silence accompanied by an evolving stare that changed from disbelief to astonishment. Sometimes, someone would offer an empathic "I'm sorry." The reality was that the rest of the world had moved on, but like the World Trade Center families, we were still figuratively at Ground Zero.

We limped into April 2003, struggling to make new identifications. We felt stuck in a rut. The families appreciated our efforts. We still felt that rush of accomplishment knowing each new identification allowed a family to move on with their lives. The hard part was that it was not happening nearly as frequently as it had a year earlier.

A rule of thumb for mass fatalities is that the last identifications are always the toughest. The data is often skimpy, family relationships are sometimes tenuous, and—as was the case in the American Airlines Flight 587 crash work, where entire families were lost—we had to identify at least one member of a family before we could find the remainder. Our experience with American Airlines Flight 587 was that 80 percent of the work went into identifying the last 20 percent of the missing. In one respect, the American Airlines Flight 587 work was easier than the World Trade Center work, because we had American Airlines's passenger manifest. As we neared the end, we knew exactly how many we still had to find. The World Trade Center work was significantly different. For most of the effort, the number of missing was a moving target. Even though Shiya finally narrowed the missing to 2,749, that number, while supposedly representing an official count, was not set in stone.

In another way, the World Trade Center work was easier than American Airlines Flight 587. The airliner crash had complex pedigrees—or family trees—that we had to sort through, complicated by entire families having been lost. The pedigree of the World Trade Center experience was simpler because the family relationships, for the most part, were not as complex, not that there were not problems. What complicated the World Trade Center work was the sheer volume of samples we had to analyze and track, poor DNA quality that led to the development of new technology, and errors that were made at the Family Assistance Centers in collecting family samples.

Once the less complex identifications had been made, these problems slowed the World Trade Center work to a crawl. Each identification required extensive piecing together of varied bits of information that included DNA, metadata, and extensive error checking. To illustrate, consider this. In June 2003, we had identified 1,508 of the missing, but by the beginning of December 2004, a year and a half later, we had identified only 77 additional people, an increase in total identifications of only 2.8 percent.

From August 2002 until December 2002, I waited impatiently for the BodePlex and SNP projects to come to fruition. Bode concluded their BodePlex developmental work and validation studies by September 2002, when they started testing remains. I hoped this signaled a new beginning. My immediate anticipation for success with degraded DNA was inextricably tied to this testing. The validation looked good, but I hoped Bode scientist Jim Schumm's redesign of the Big Mini concept would be successful.

I was of two minds about our chances of success. My emotional side prayed BodePlex would spawn an avalanche of new identifications. My scientific side, however, had reservations. We were working with our backs against the wall. I certainly knew that many who died had been buried in the hottest part of the World Trade Center rubble; anyone who had been watching the evening news for the first months of the rescue-recovery effort had seen the smoke and heard about the intense heat. We might never identify those poor souls, even if we had found them. I was hoping for new identifications but was expecting to find more pieces of people we already knew about. While not bad, it was not the ideal or what I really wanted.

Our first BodePlex data arrived in MFISys on December 20, 2002. We had 5 new identifications! It was a grand day. The sobering part was that these 5 gave us a grand total of 8 for the entire month. Still, it was a huge emotional lift. Everyone on the second floor was wearing broad, expectant smiles, and there were high fives all around. Elaine sent an e-mail to the entire laboratory announcing the success. I guardedly anticipated a return to the halcyon days of the past spring and summer, when we were making upwards of a hundred new identifications a month.

New identifications rose from 8 in December to 11 in January 2003. I prayed we were once again on the right track. After so many nervous months of waiting and praying that the miniplex concept would work, especially after the Big Mini disappointment of a year earlier, my decision to embark on a second miniplex project with Bode had been justified. We had made identifications that we could not have made just a day earlier. There was no reason to expect that would change.

Then the rise in new identifications faltered: February and March had 10 and 13, respectively; April had 6, and May, only 5. It was a tough time for us all. In retrospect, I suppose I should never have let my hopes soar. BodePlex had been designed to add data to partial-STR profiles. In reality, BodePlex, or any miniplex for that matter, could not be expected to work magic on the vast number of DMs that had given no STR results after two phases of DNA testing. The World Trade Center epitaph for BodePlex might read something like this: a novel technique that successfully identified many who perished where other techniques had failed, and proved invaluable in re-associating remains of people who had already been identified.

What about those remains whose DNA was even more degraded? Would we ever make identifications from those? I harbored hope.

The first two phases of STR testing ended with approximately 28 percent of the remains yielding no STR results. A significant percentage of these had given either complete or partial mitochondrial DNA mitotypes, which meant usable mtDNA was present. Although mitotypes alone are not sufficient to make identifications, this knowledge led me to formulate a follow-on contract with a company called Affymetrix to develop a method for DNA sequencing the entire mitochondrial DNA genome. Unfortunately, that technology, if it proved successful on World Trade Center samples, would not be ready for three years. For the short term, I counted on SNPs.

Orchid finally completed its SNP validation in April 2003. I received the data from Bob Giles and hoped it represented the last of the experiments. The study included work on 961 DMs that Lydia had sent to the company in March. Orchid had to demonstrate that it could obtain consistent test results on a blind set of triplicate DMs specifically chosen to represent the vast array of degraded DNAs we had encountered. It was the final KADAP validation experiment.

I downloaded Bob Giles's file, a series of spreadsheets, and then nervously studied the data. I desperately wanted the data to show what I wanted. I warned myself that I could not be biased. I also had to steel myself for disappointment.

Bob had grouped the DMs based on their SNP profiles. If the validation meant I was going forward with SNP typing on DMs, these SNP groups had to match the known STR groups. Bob had not had access to the STR profiles. As I scanned the spreadsheet from top to bottom, my first thought was, Okay, this looks encouraging.

I reworked the data, grouping the DMs by STRs, and then compared those groups with Orchid's SNP groups. I was looking for consistency. If it was there, it meant SNPs could be used for the World Trade Center DNA work. If it wasn't, SNPs would be out of the picture. My heart was beating faster as I compared the two data groups. If they did not match up, I would have a lot of explaining to do to the press and to Chuck Hirsch.

They matched.

Orchid had completed the SNP validation successfully. Before putting the test online, I needed someone to agree with my assessment. I had to schedule a meeting in Dallas, where a separate group of scientists would review the data and, I hoped, agree. I also had to review Orchid's sample-handling processes to ensure that the company was maintaining appropriate control of the samples.

Forming this independent group of scientists turned out to be easier said than done. My preference would have been to have scientists from the KADAP review the data and then sign off on it. However, the panel, which had worked tirelessly in the initial SNP validation work and with the BodePlex validation and also with the mtDNA validation to its completion, had decided that it no longer could be involved.

This left me high and dry. I turned to other scientists who would give an independent, objective opinion about the data. Charles Brenner, a nongovernment member of the KADAP, and Dr. Ranajit Chakraborty, a professor at the University of Cincinnati, agreed to help.

My next problem was scheduling. I wanted the meeting in Dallas scheduled as soon as possible, ideally before the end of April, but the first week in May was the earliest mutually convenient time. And it would have to be at the end of the week because I had agreed to speak before a high school class in Allentown, Pennsylvania, about the World Trade Center work that Wednesday.

Howard Baum and I left for Dallas on Thursday. I was exhausted and feeling the pressure, not just because of the World Trade Center work but also because of my schedule. I needed to relax, but that was impossible, even on the plane, where I normally have no trouble sleeping, especially when I was that tired.

The next morning, we met at Orchid, got a quick tour of their facilities, and then met in the conference room to review the SNP data. I was guarded. I had held out so much hope that this would be the panacea for degraded World Trade Center DNA. Of the scientists with me, only Ranajit had not been involved with the KADAP. Although the others were members of the panel, they were not federal employees, so they could work with me. Ranajit was the only one who did not have a vested interest in the work. At the end of the second day, we agreed that the SNP data appeared sound. From my perspective, the meeting went well. There was no reason that SNP testing on DMs should be delayed any longer. Now it was a matter of waiting to see how successful the technique would be.

After Dallas, I was off to Florida. The first three days of the next week, the week of May 12, I spoke at the Second Annual Bode Advanced DNA Workshop at the Hawk's Cay Resort on Duck Key in the Florida Keys. My presentation on Tuesday centered on lessons learned from the World Trade Center work.

My schedule had finally caught up with me. It had been a grueling couple of months, and I was dead tired. I had no trouble convincing Fran to spend the remainder of the week relaxing in Key West. The Hawk's Cay Resort on Duck Key is only about an hour's drive east of Key West, so it was an easy trip.

Key West, the southernmost point in the continental United States, is a place everyone should experience at least once in a lifetime. It's a funky, fun place set in a tropical paradise. This was our second visit there, and we stayed at the Heron House again, an elegant bed-and-breakfast. The B&B is located within walking distance of most every tourist attraction in the area, especially the main drag, Duval Street, and the nice, albeit expensive, restaurants there. This would be our only time off since the week before September 11.

Relaxing for two days on Key West sounded like a welcome prescription for someone who was pretty much burned out. We arrived, unpacked, and then strolled up and down Duval Street, soaked in the heat and sun, had a couple of margaritas in Jimmy Buffett's Margaritaville restaurant, bought a couple of Margaritaville T-shirts, and ate well.

Fran wanted to see the lunar eclipse, so we booked a tour on the tourist schooner the *America*, which was the winning schooner of the first America's Cup race in 1851, where it defeated fourteen British schooners. That night, though, the captain never raised the sails—claiming time restraint and the nighttime danger. I would have liked to have cruised under sail, but we did see the eclipse anyhow.

The alternative was to wedge among the hundreds of other vacationers jockeying for position on the Mallory Square pier, which I thought would be too much like fighting Times Square crowds in New York.

The next evening we decided on a sunset cruise and chose the last floating World War II PT boat, PT-728, a testosterone high for sure. I secured a spot in the machine gun turret, which was great fun. Saturday arrived too soon. It was time to leave the tropics and head home. Key West had been the perfect pause; no responsibilities and no hectic schedule. To be honest, though, being away from the city had made me anxious. I felt out of touch, and I never really divorced myself completely from my work. The two days had passed too quickly, and I felt like I should have stayed another week, but I needed to get back to work.

I had just completed packing and was lifting the suitcase from the bed to the floor when I felt a sharp, persistent pain in the center of my chest unlike any I had experienced before. It is difficult to describe it exactly, but it was intense and growing. I braced myself and stood still a moment to see if it would pass. It didn't.

A cold sweat formed on my head and forehead. I felt nauseous, and my skin quickly turned cold and clammy. I laid on the bed and tried to will my body to relax, wishing the pain away. Certainly this will pass, I thought.

Then I began sweating profusely. In seconds I was drenched. By now, the pain was sucking away my breath and my strength. It was un-relenting, a growing, burning epicenter inside my chest. Then a dull ache developed in the bicep of my left arm. I knew what was happening.

I always feared I would die from a massive coronary, as my father did when I was only four. I kept telling myself, Don't move. I sensed if I did anything physical, I would die.

I felt weak, and I wondered if I could even stand. When I think back on it, I wonder whether I even had the strength to operate my cell phone, or if I had, would such little activity have killed me. One thought surfaced, Was this the same pain my father felt before he died?

Fran came out of the bathroom seconds after I lay down on the bed, and saw me. She sat on the bed beside me. "Are you all right?" she asked.

I was purposefully taking very shallow breaths, and I was having trouble speaking. I tried to explain what was happening. "Should I call a doctor?" she asked. I nodded and whispered, "Yes."

Now it was a race against time, and I knew it. Was it my turn? A myriad of thoughts flooded my mind. One stuck: Please, God, I have too much more to do.

• • •

Sunday June 22, 2003, was raining, overcast, and about 60 degrees when we arrived at the intersection of 30th Avenue and 87th Street in Jackson Heights, Queens, a little after 10:00 A.M.

I had been a patient in three hospitals. The first was the emergency room in Key West, followed closely by Mount Sinai in Miami, Florida, and NYU Medical Center in New York. I now had three stents in two of my coronary arteries. A month after my heart attack, I was feeling strong. I had lost weight, which felt really good. The forced "vacation" had me feeling relaxed for the first time in almost two years.

Fran and I arrived early. I asked two official-looking men who stood in the street near the corner where we could park. "Drive down the street and take anything you can find," one said. Then he motioned to a tiny space behind a black SUV at the corner. "You can probably fit there."

I steered my Toyota MR2 Spyder behind the SUV, getting as close to his bumper as I could without hitting it. I looked up at the 87th Street sign and saw another sign wrapped in paper under it. I assumed the paper was hiding James's name.

A couple of minutes later, I spied John Cartier wearing a dark brown leather Australian-style hat, a Local 103 black vest, his hair braided into a long ponytail, walking purposefully toward the corner. A number of the IBEW Motorcycle Club bikes were parked on 30th Avenue.

He spotted me; I got out of the car and met him in the middle of 87th Street. Our hands met as though to shake, but we hugged instead. It was good to see him. It had been a long time, like forever. I really like this man, a gentle soul wrapped in a solid body. John looked me in the eyes and said, "How are you feeling?"

"Great," I replied. John's question wasn't the usual casual "How're ya doin'?" It felt different. His eyes were searching, his face questioning. It was the first time we had seen each other since my heart attack. Many that morning expressed their concern, especially the Cartiers. Even those who had lost loved ones who had not yet been identified were genuinely glad to see me.

Minutes later, the corner began filling with people. Several men wore kilts and carried bagpipe cases, which they began unpacking, and then they warmed up their instruments, issuing discordant sounds that pierced the air. It was both harsh but pleasing and strangely melodious without a song being played.

By 10:30, the rain was still a constant drizzle. The sky was gray but not ominously dark. The air felt cool but not uncomfortable. I saw Jennie, got out of the car, and approached her. When she saw me, her expression matched John's, a mixture of concern and joy. Seeing her was also cathartic. We held each other for a few seconds. A couple of minutes later, Michele Cartier and I embraced.

By now about fifty people were milling around, exchanging greetings. I heard a smattering of laughter, pockets of which popped up almost sporadically. Lengthy embraces were common. A few minutes before the ceremony began, James's sister Marie and her husband, Mike, joined the group. I made a point to say hello. She too had lost a lot of weight and looked terrific. We held each other tightly for some time, just as I did with James's brother Mike when he arrived with his family.

Several people—some of their names I remembered and others I did not, although I did recognize their faces—made a point to shake my hand and wish me well. Katie and Francis Sullivan and Shiya and his wife, Jen, arrived, followed by scientists from my lab: Noelle Umback, Bianca Nazzaurolo, and Sheila Estacio. Naturally, Howard Cash showed up, too. A woman with sad brown eyes whom I knew but whose name I could not remember stood next to me shielding herself with an umbrella. She grasped my upper arm in her hand. "I see you identified three more," she said, referring to new identifications reported in the newspaper.

It was a statement of hope, I realized. We had not yet identified her son.

I said, "We are still working to identify everyone." I had experienced this scene with dozens of families. Each time I felt inadequate.

Her eyes said she understood. "I know," she said. "We all thank you." She turned and walked away.

Eventually, more than one hundred people showed up to celebrate changing the name of James's boyhood street from 87th Street to James Marcel Cartier Way. James would have been twenty-eight, but the Cartiers considered this his second birthday—his first was a year earlier at his funeral, when we buried his remains.

Jennie walked to a microphone and asked for everyone's attention. She welcomed us, then gave an emotional presentation. Bagpipers played "America the Beautiful," a priest gave a benediction, we pledged allegiance to the flag, and then Jennie's cousin Gary sang an inspired "Star-Spangled Banner."

Richie Scherer, the Office of Emergency Management director on September 11, represented Mayor Giuliani and said a few words. Governor Pataki's representative, Tara Snow, read a letter written by the governor. Jennie read another letter written by James's brothers and sisters for their parents. Gary sang a song written by Michele, after which it was time to unwrap the new street sign. The Cartier family gathered around and tugged on the rope. As the paper fell way, the new white letters on the dark green background gleamed. The sign read JAMES MARCEL CARTIER WAY. Everyone was in tears.

It was still raining five minutes before the ceremony was slated to begin at 11:00 A.M. When Jennie placed her hand on the microphone a few minutes before 11:00 the rain stopped, the sky miraculously cleared and turned a beautiful light azure with puffy white clouds. The ceremony lasted only about a half hour and the sun shone brightly throughout. I stood next to James's oldest brother, Patrick, who looked skyward and said, "James is with us."

I had goose bumps. It reminded me of the first September 11 anniversary, when the strong wind had kicked up a dust cloud. The spirits of those who died had been with us at the World Trade Center site, just as James was with us that Sunday.

26 FINALLY ... SNPs

May 31, 2004
Missing Identified: 1,552
DNA Identifications: 812

On September 8, 2003, I received a letter dated August 26 from the chairperson of the New York City Department of Health Institutional Review Board addressing our application to make World Trade Center identifications using SNPs.

After reading the letter I had to smile. It seemed a bit late for the city to begin enforcing federal regulations to grant the city (actually the OCME) permission to do something it had been doing for almost two years. In reality, it was a hoop we needed to jump through to avoid future criticism. Frankly, too, I believe it was also a cover-your-butt response and the culmination of almost a year's effort to comply with suggestions made at an early KADAP meeting.

The ruling meant I was permitted to use SNPs to make identifications. Unfortunately, there was still a problem. As far as the New York State Department of Health was concerned, I was not supposed to use SNPs to make identifications until Dr. Anne Walsh signed off on the Orchid validation. It seemed like a hopelessly tangled mess. On one hand, I needed Institutional Review Board approval and on the other, I needed the New York State Department of Health approval. The Institutional Review Board approval, however, was a step in the right direction.

The Institutional Review Board has the responsibility of approving all New York City government–sponsored biological research involving living subjects in the City of New York. Its basic role is to ensure that there is "informed consent" for those who are the subjects of biological research. Researchers must complete a complicated application spelling out, in part, exactly what will be done, who will participate, how informed consent will be obtained, and the expected outcome of the research. Since the World Trade Center identification effort had been funded by FEMA, a federal agency, our identification efforts supposedly fell within the purview of the city's Institutional Review Board.

Each institution (e.g., each university or hospital) has its own institutional review board that acts independently. Each institutional review board is tasked to apply federal guidelines. Since each institutional review board is independent from all others, one institutional review board might sanction a specific project while another might not. There is little consistency among these boards.

At a fall 2002 KADAP meeting, the National Institutes of Health members of the panel had an epiphany. They suddenly thought or remembered that the DNA part of our World Trade Center identification work, especially with respect to "new" technology, fell under federal guidelines. This meant I needed Institutional Review Board approval to use the new technology to make identifications. It was a problem. If true, it meant the OCME (me) had been in violation of federal law. Although I seriously doubted the feds would close down the OCME—imagine the public outcry—I faced the real and troubling possibility it could happen. My main concern was losing the advice and expertise of the panel scientists; as we neared the end of the project, I felt their expertise with difficult identifications might be invaluable.

By city charter, the OCME has the obligation to investigate suspicious deaths in the City of New York and to identify—name— bodies associated with those deaths. This is work performed in the agency's routine course of business. The OCME does not require Institutional Review Board approval to perform its city charter-mandated mission. Imagine the mess if the OCME had to apply for and wait for Institutional Review Board approval to identify everyone who died in the city—approximately 70,000 annually. Certainly, the deaths resulting from the terrorist attacks on the World Trade Center were murders. As such, they clearly fell within the OCME's mission. The problem had to do with the technology I planned to employ.

But why SNPs as opposed to the other validation testing? Actually, the original KADAP concern included all of what they referred to as the World Trade Center "research projects." This included miniplexes and SNPs. However, when the OCME approached the Institutional Review Board in July and August 2003, the BodePlex work for the World Trade Center effort was virtually complete. The federal scientists on the KADAP politely refused to review the final Bode validation data for BodePlex, so Howard Baum and I went to Bode in September 2002 to review the data. Interestingly, the same Institutional Review Board concern never came up when John Butler did his validation for the Big Mini in December 2001 and January 2002. At the time, I doubt the KADAP scientists had even considered the Institutional Review Board. We were working through a number of pressing DNA issues, although my plan to pursue SNP and miniplex technologies had not been kept secret.

The first mention of Institutional Review Board approval came up during a conference call of the KADAP SNP subgroup meeting, probably in the summer of 2002. I don't specifically recall who from the National Institutes of Health group first mentioned it, but once the topic had been broached, the NIH folks became concerned that the SNP and the miniplex projects fell under the federal regulations and required Institutional Review Board approval. They made it abundantly clear that they would have nothing to do with any discussion concerning SNPs.

I was shocked. I am pretty naïve, maybe a bit old-fashioned, but I always thought scientists pursued science because it was, well, science. It bothered me that highly trained scientists and well-intentioned people would abdicate a responsibility for something as simple as applying a new technology to a pressing scientific problem. At the very least, I would have expected them to continue working toward the final end. This is not what happened. I wanted their input, so I had no choice but to acquiesce to their concerns and raise the Institutional Review Board issue to my boss, Chuck Hirsch. Before this, I had little experience with institutional review boards, except to know that such regulations existed and that the OCME had to comply with the federal regulations when planning to do research involving human subjects.

Chuck opined that all the World Trade Center work fell within the OCME's mission to identify bodies in New York City deaths. He articulated that the OCME did not need to apply for Institutional Review Board approval to use DNA testing to identify World Trade Center victims. Neither of us believed we were performing research on living subjects, although we had taken samples from family members to use in kinship analyses. Needless to say, his logic did not satisfy the National Institutes of Health or the other federal Kinship and Data Analysis Panel scientists. We were at an impasse. I was in danger of losing a potentially valuable resource.

The Institutional Review Board topic came up again at the final regularly scheduled KADAP meeting in July 2003. The National Institutes of Health scientists would not help make identifications on potential identifications requiring SNPs unless I obtained Institutional Review Board approval.

I approached Chuck again about the problem. This time, I also mentioned the issue of needing the New York State Department of Health to sign off on the SNP validation data.

Dr. Anne Walsh was waiting for Orchid to reply to her request to review the final validation work. The problem is that she wanted the KADAP to sign off on SNPs, which I believe would have made her feel more comfortable about a technology with which she was not that familiar. I felt she wanted to wait for the panel to pass on SNPs before she passed on Orchid analyzing World Trade Center DMs, although she had already agreed to allow the company to analyze family buccal swabs.

I reminded her that the KADAP was only an advisory group and did not have policy-making power and that neither the OCME nor the New York State Department of Health required the panel to sign off on SNPs before blessing the technology. She understood that. I also pointed out that this is exactly what happened with the Bode-Plex validation studies. She had signed off on that technology. I hinted that the Institutional Review Board approval process might be lengthy, which meant holding off using SNP technology for making identifications, which would have been an additional delay, and which I felt was unsatisfactory. Anne agreed with my logic, but I felt she had not been convinced. I believed she was uncomfortable with the technology and was looking for support.

Shortly after the second September 11 anniversary date in 2003, when I spoke to her about moving SNPs online and told her about the Institutional Review Board approval problem, she expressed several legitimate concerns. First, the technology generated what we called "failures." This meant there were no results obtained on some SNPs where they were expected. Failures occurred by one of two mechanisms, either because of degraded DNA or because there had been too little DNA extract to obtain an SNP type. Anne wanted Orchid to devise a mechanism for determining why a particular SNP failed. She believed this would be a nice addition to any future study using SNPs to type badly degraded samples. Though I did not disagree in principle, I believed that withholding SNP testing on the DMs in order to conduct a study that could not be done easily or might even be impossible at that time was unnecessary. A failed SNP meant no results with which to make a comparison, which would affect the matching statistics, regardless of whether it happened because of degraded DNA or too little DNA in the reaction vessel.

I was partially wrong. True, a failure affected the matching statistics, but why the failure occurred could have far-reaching consequences with respect to interpreting the reliability of the SNP test results.

Because of the meeting I had in Dallas, the SNP work had already begun on DMs without New York State Department of Health approval. Backtracking to answer Anne's concern would have meant reextracting thousands of DMs, which would have delayed us months. The project was already dragging my staff down, and to ask the sixth-floor disaster team to reextract the original DMs for the fourth time would have been unfair and, I felt, unnecessary. Lydia would have glared at me for a moment, moved her head from side to side as only she can, and then would have said, "You want to what?" Then, as she sharpened her verbal knife before beheading me, she would have said, "Do you know how many weeks that would take?"

Meanwhile, the SNP data was streaming into the lab.

On December 11, 2003, we had our first SNP identification. I was at home recovering from a broken ankle and nose, the result of a fall during a testosterone-induced renovation project at a condo Fran and I bought in November 2003 in Dewey Beach, Delaware. My accident occurred three days before Thanksgiving—great timing—and I was under strict doctor's orders to stay off my leg. E-mails from Elaine Mar kept me abreast of the World Trade Center work, and Howard Baum was giving me running tabs on overall lab work via cell phone.

Elaine had been working on a new identification where the match included a partial STR profile from a personal effect that matched a DM. The match looked good, but the statistics fell short of the KADAP threshold, although we also had a mito match. Still, she was reluctant to call it.

I asked her to scan the data and e-mail it to me so I could examine it, which she did. I wanted to check the STR electropherograms myself, although there was really no reason to question her interpretation except to keep myself busy and to convince myself that there was no additional data available that might be used to make the identification. Truthfully, the second-floor DNA identification group was probably better at examining the data than I because they saw more of it, but I still wanted to check it for myself. I suppose I was hoping against hope to find something they had missed. I checked the electropherograms. We were not going to make the identification using STRs. It was a sad realization, but only one of many we had run across the past two years.

Then, on December 11, I received an e-mail titled, "First SNP ID." I was shocked to see that it was the same RM. Since I had reviewed the electropherograms, new SNP data had come from Gene Codes Forensics for both the DM and for the personal effect. They matched, and the statistics exceeded the KADAP recommendations by twentyfold.

There was still a nagging problem, though. Anne had not given Orchid the go-ahead, a fact I wrestled with for the remainder of the day. I knew the science was good, so it was really a political problem, one I thought might come back in the future and kick me in the butt. Politics aside, how could I, in good conscience, hold back an identification when I saw no valid scientific reason to do so? I instructed Elaine to report the identification.

During the SNP validation, mismatches had become a sticky part of interpreting SNP data.

I went to the Third Annual National Institute of Justice Grantees conference in June 2002, where recipients of National Institute of Justice forensic research grants presented the results of their research to representatives from each crime lab in the United States. Lisa Forman had asked me to give a talk on the World Trade Center work, and I convinced her to invite the Cartiers to speak. I believed that that wonderful family could provide some insight for these scientists who rarely experienced the emotional consequences of their work.

At a break, Mandy Sozer, Steve Niezgoda, Lisa Forman, and I spent an hour working out the logistics of the KADAP SNP subpanel scheduled to meet the next Tuesday, July 2. The subpanel was supposed to make recommendations to the KADAP, but there was a scheduling problem related to funding. Also, the SNP validation had been dragging on, and Lisa was beginning to believe Orchid would never satisfy the KADAP.

She asked me, "What is your final line in the sand?" She was asking for the date when I would agree to cut off Orchid if their validation dragged on much longer. She was also referring to my statement to the KADAP—and to the contract laboratories—with respect to the mayor's suggestion to complete the bulk of DNA testing on DMs by the anniversary date in September 2002.

In fact, Mayor Michael Bloomberg had never specifically said, "I want the work finished by the anniversary." However, on a tour through the DNA lab soon after he took office, he did ask, "When do you think DNA testing will be completed?"

"I hope by the anniversary," I had replied, knowing there was better than a 50–50 chance I would be proven wrong.

He was walking in front of me. He turned and said, "That would be appropriate."

I used this response to prod—"goose"—the contract laboratories into believing it was a mayoral directive when it really was not.

Lisa wanted a decision. As I sat there searching for words to hedge, I was reminded of the day in February when Steve Niezgoda asked me to commit to a time line of target dates for completing DNA testing.

As though reading my mind, she said, "This is the third date drawn in the sand for SNPs." She hesitated. "What if they aren't ready?"

A bogus mayoral anniversary deadline or not, I really did not want to abandon SNP testing without seeing how it worked with DMs. I had been telling Chuck Hirsch and the families that SNPs would be our last line of testing. I wanted to give the technology a chance. If it failed, so be it. I could live with that. But I was having trouble choosing an arbitrary date to cut off the validation work without having more validation data. In truth, I was not about to cut them off. Not yet.

"It's a moving line," I said, poker-faced. "If Orchid's capacity is truly what they say it is, then they can still make the September 11 stop-testing date, even if they start in August." I had no idea whether this was true or not, but it sounded good.

Lisa's expression belied her words. "Okay, so we work with them."

The next KADAP meeting was scheduled for July 11, 2002. Presumably, I was to receive Orchid's validation data on the ninth, which would be followed by a conference call on the tenth with the SNP subpanel.

I said, "If the subpanel suggests more validation, we can take a closer look at Orchid's sample tracking and make sure they have everything in place when they are ready to start. Also, Howard Cash won't be ready to accept SNPs into MFISys until August . . . so, I have time." I continued, "Ideally, the Kinship and Data Analysis Panel blesses Orchid's validation study, which will make it easier for Anne Walsh to sign off on Orchid." Lisa nodded.

Then someone called to Lisa, so she had to return to the meeting. I left to work on my presentation scheduled for the next morning, but ran into Randy Nagy, Bode's vice president of marketing, who invited me to go across the street to Murphy's DC for a beer. How could I pass up the invitation?

SNPs represented a new adventure in testing for forensic scientists. No public or private crime laboratory in the United States employed them for everyday criminal casework, let alone to perform genetic analysis on such badly compromised samples. In forensic terms, the World Trade Center SNP project was huge. Aside from perhaps the Armed Forces DNA Identification Lab and National Institute of Science and Technology, federal agencies doing research on mitochondrial SNPs and discussions about SNPs among forensic DNA scientists before September 11 were few and far between.

For much of the World Trade Center work, especially in the beginning, I had looked to the FBI for help. Mostly, I felt the bureau had abandoned me. In the area of SNPs, however, the FBI's Dr. Bruce Budowle, a research scientist, turned out to be one of my staunchest supporters. He understood the World Trade Center program and my needs as well as anyone, and he never failed to voice a favorable opinion at KADAP meetings when I thought the panel was on the verge of recommending canceling the World Trade Center SNP effort.

There are good reasons why forensic scientists have not embraced SNPs. First, individually, SNPs do not have as great an ability to make specific identifications as STRs. In order to reach the statistical threshold of the 13 CODIS STRs, one would have to type approximately 40 SNPs, a higher analytical burden. Also, the testing format would have to be adapted to the instrumentation used in U.S. crime laboratories, which would require a new set of interpretation standards. It would be a steep learning curve.

When I embarked on a quest to use SNPs for World Trade Center DNA identifications, I was wading into uncharted waters. I needed help, and I knew it. The KADAP reviewed the first SNP data in February 2002, when Dr. Bob Giles presented the first of Orchid's validation data. I remember feeling anxious. However, as he spoke, I saw merit in my decision to move forward with the technology. I also realized the test needed a lot of work. The panel agreed. During a break, Bob confided privately that he believed SNPs might be ready by the June deadline. It was wishful thinking. Howard Baum expressed his doubts. He was correct.

The panel formed an SNP subpanel that met on July 12, 2002, in Washington, DC. Lisa and Mandy rounded up a group of scientists who had SNP experience, many of whom were panel members, others who were not. The subcommittee's task was to consider SNPs as a potential tool to make identifications for the World Trade Center effort. At this first meeting, Bob Giles and Dr. Jeanine Baiche, also of Orchid, presented their work, which they hoped would convince the KADAP once and for all that SNPs were ready for the World Trade Center effort. I suspect the Orchid folks expected to walk away from the meeting with an endorsement. It did not come.

The subcommittee correctly concluded that Orchid had to do

additional work and suggested several experiments. I agreed with the panel's decision, but again I saw promise. Orchid's work on compromised samples looked enticing. They had obtained results where STRs had not. I guess the KADAP members saw the same promise I did or they would have recommended canceling the program.

The main problem with SNPs was the high failure rate. Over time, I learned more about the characteristics of individual SNPs. One of the biggest problems was knowing when a test result was reliable. The original test devised by Orchid was so sensitive that many SNPs gave results even when there was almost no DNA remaining. With declining amounts of DNA, a particular SNP would give a consistent result and then, at some low concentration of DNA, give a completely different one. This was upsetting because it left open the possibility that a test result was incorrect, a mismatch, without a way of knowing it. This happened with low levels of target DNA, which was particularly relevant to the World Trade Center work because a high percentage of the DMs had low levels of DNA.

Orchid discovered a group of SNPs it called threshold SNPs, or TSNPs. These TSNPs were hardy, meaning they generally gave reliable results until they failed, without an intermediary incorrect result. When these TSNPs failed, the general complexion of the resulting SNP profiles also deteriorated. This was the point at which other, nonhardy SNPs tended to give unreliable test results. This information pointed us toward a mechanism for determining the reliability of SNP data.

If all of the TSNPs gave a positive test result, we felt confident that the other SNP tests were valid. However, once a TSNP failed, we felt that the reliability of the data had to be questioned because experience had shown that the number of mismatches increased. After examining hundreds of SNP profiles, however, I learned that TSNPs were not necessarily a hard-and-fast dividing line between good and bad SNP data. I regularly found SNP profiles where all four of the TSNPs had failed, but there were no mismatches to, say, a personal effect with other SNPs. We decided we had to interpret all SNP profiles carefully, even those without failed TSNPs, if there were mismatches.

TABLE 6: SNP INTERPRETATIONS

SAMPLE	NO. STRs	NO. SNPs	NO. FAILED TSNPs	NO. MISMATCHES
Personal Effect 1	14	62	0	0
Personal Effect 2	12	58	1	0
DM 1	10	71	0	1
DM 2	6	70	0	0
DM 3	0	46	1	0
DM 4	5	45	3	2
DM 5	4	33	3	2
DM 6	0	32	3	3

For Table 6, I chose an RM (reported missing person) in a group sorted according to matching SNP profiles. Where there are STR profiles, they also matched. The second column shows the number of STRs obtained for a particular personal effect or DM. The third column is the number of SNPs obtained (out of a possible 71) for a personal effect or DM, the fourth column is the number of failed TSNPs for each personal effect or DM, and the last column is the number of mismatches, where mismatches represent differences between the personal effect and the DM SNP profiles.

The personal effects in the top two rows are from the same missing person. They have 14 and 12 STRs respectively and 62 and 58 SNPs respectively. The lower PE has one failed TSNP (shaded) but no mismatches when compared to the PE above. Since these personal effects come from the same person, we expected a perfect match, meaning no mismatches. The single failed TSNP has no consequence because there are no mismatches.

The number of SNPs obtained for the DMs range from 32 to 71 and were cross-referenced with 0 to 10 STRs.

The number of failed TSNPs, the fourth column, generally correlates with the number of mismatches, fifth column, which is what Orchid found in their initial validation experiments. However, this isn't always true, and having failed TSNPs does not necessarily mean that the data is unusable. For DM 3, the 1 failed TSNP for the 46 SNPs correlated to no mismatches. This is usable data.

However, as the number of TSNPs increased, the number of mismatches also increased, especially as the total number of SNPs decreased, the number of mismatches increased. This is what is seen for DMs 4, 5, and 6 (dark shaded area), where the number of mismatches (black shading) is unacceptable.

The point is that generalities are guidelines and not necessarily diagnostic for specific situations. Each SNP match had to be analyzed on its own merits, and we made determinations on whether the data were valid and the calculations sufficiently reliable to make a match. In the above example, the mismatches were caused by allelic dropout. Like STRs, allelic dropout with SNPs was not unexpected.

The unexpected surprise with SNPs was the finding that mismatches occurred with the same DM tested multiple times. That is, the same sample gave presumably different SNP profiles! This is illustrated in the table above with the two PEs (top two rows). Their profiles, though mostly matching, are exact matches. Mismatches such as these were particularly disconcerting because it meant that DMs originating from the same person might appear to come from different people, when they should be identical. I quickly learned that mismatches happen for varying reasons and were not necessarily fatal. As I studied the data and began to understand why they occurred, I realized that they were not as damaging with respect to making a final determination of reliability as I had originally thought.

After several experiments, Bob and Jeanine concluded that two

DMs came from the same person if no more than 5 percent of the SNPs in a profile did not match, provided that a sufficient number of SNPs gave results. Admittedly, this was a ballpark estimate, but it confirmed what I had been seeing as I explored the data. I preferred a more rigorous approach. I asked Charles Brenner to devise a mathematical expression that would allow us to calculate the likelihood ratios, given mismatches. The question I was really asking was, how many mismatches could I tolerate before declaring that two samples were not from the same source? I did not have his first attempt at the problem until October 2003, which he then revised in January 2004.

A third problem surfaced during a KADAP meeting when, after examining genetic maps of the SNP panel proposed by Orchid, Steve Sherry and Elizabeth Pugh pointed out that most of those chosen by Orchid were linked, although Ranajit Chakraborty, a respected geneticist at the University of Cincinnati, had examined Orchid's SNP data and wrote a report that differed, from a practical sense. Still, it appeared to be a concern. Charles also disagreed. He expressed his opinion that it did not affect our ability to use SNPs to make direct matches.

A fourth problem reflected Howard Baum's original concern with mixtures, the reason why he originally believed SNPs would never work. This was important because, for example, if two DMs shared the same but partial STR profile, I needed to confirm that they both came from the same person. If one of the samples had been commingled either after the buildings collapsed or during the recovery process, the SNP testing might reflect the composite of both deceased people. From a practical perspective, the two DM SNP profiles would not match. After examining hundreds of SNP profiles separated into groups by STR type, I figured out a way to identify a mixture, but only if the DM or PE had a nearly complete SNP profiles. Those having partial SNP profiles were not amenable to this kind of examination.

Orchid ended up with a panel of 71 SNP loci, one of which was the sexing gene, and we eventually tested all the DNA extracts from DMs, personal effects, and family kinship samples.

27 QUALITY ASSURANCE

December 31, 2003

Quality assurance data in MFISys:

DMs STR typed more than once: 12,940

DMs with consistent STR profiles: 11,356

Conflicts yet to be resolved: 146

Resolved conflicts: 1,438

The call from Howard Cash to me in Florida in February 2002 alerted me to the first instance of a growing problem I had to tackle: conflicting DNA profiles.

So, once the September 2001 chaos clamed down, I had to think seriously about resolving them.

Coincidentally, Larry Quarino, a professor of forensic science at Cedar Crest College in Pennsylvania, called about a summer position that might be available. Larry had worked in my laboratory as a supervising criminalist but resigned after receiving his PhD from the City University of New York (CUNY). His first job after the OCME was an abbreviated sojourn at a university in California, after which he accepted the position at Cedar Crest. I immediately hired him and asked him to establish a quality-assurance monitoring program for the World Trade Center work. His call could not have been more perfectly timed. I needed someone to resolve STR conflicts, but it had to be someone familiar with STRs in a forensic context. Larry fit the bill perfectly, and hiring him meant I would not be taking my own scientists out of the laboratory, which could have disrupted the routine homicide and sexual-assault casework.

When I spoke to Larry, I thought that resolving the STR conflicts would be relatively simple. I naïvely thought it would be a matter of reviewing the conflicting data, finding the problem, and resolving it. I incorrectly thought that the vast majority of these conflicts would be examples of commingled remains or allelic dropout. Certainly, I anticipated an occasional mixed-up sample.

By the end of the summer, Larry had established a protocol to resolve the conflicts and was working through the data to find and resolve them. This was a time-consuming process. Larry left at the end of summer 2002, when it was time for him to resume his teaching responsibilities. Erik Bieschke took over.

Resolving these problems often required retesting. The special projects group worked on most of them. Sometimes the sixth-floor disaster team sent the DMs to Bode. For example, if a bone and a tissue had the same DM number but different STR profiles, the best and simplest way to resolve the problem or to prove that there really was a problem was to retest. Either Amy Mundorff or Zoran Budimlija would go to Memorial Park and resample the original remains.

I expected such retesting would mimic the original STR results, which meant that the DMs came from different people, meaning that the STR testing resulted from the commingling. This was completely explainable given the mechanism by which the buildings fell and people died together. We documented these findings to our satisfaction.

After resampling, Amy would "split" the DMs, which meant she voided the original "core" number (the number assigned to remains as they were received into the OCME morgue) and gave each separated piece a new "core" number, so that they were now no longer considered a part of the same DM. In essence, she converted the bone and tissue, which had shared a DM number, into two different DM numbers. We called these split cases.

We learned that poor-quality DNA was another and more common reason why STR profiles differed. As I have already discussed, decomposing DMs often gave DNA profiles that seemed like full profiles but in reality were not. Often, the conflicts showed up only after multiple testing of the same DM, as DM testing moved from Phase I to Phase III. The most prevalent example of this was allelic dropout. An STR profile from a DM and its retest might give data like that shown in Table 7.

TABLE 7. ALLELIC DROPOUT

DM Analysis 1	XY	14/16	17	12/13	28/29	10/11	11/12	13	8/9	13
DM Analysis 2	XY	14/16	17	12/13	28/29	10/11	11/12	10/13	8/9	10

The DMs in Table 7 above have the same core number, which means the ME who removed them from the remains believed they came from the same missing person and assigned them the same DM number. The DM might be as simple as a piece of bone with attached tissue. The ME would sample the bone and the tissue, usually not even separating them, and put them into the same collection tube. After STR analysis, the results showed up in MFISys in the format shown above.

This example shows STR results at 10 loci. A quick glance at the profiles individually would not raise the suspicion that anything was wrong. However, since both have the same core DM number, the results should be identical. They are not, which meant we had to find out why. This was Larry's job.

The samples are from a male, as shown by the XY test result. Seven other loci match perfectly, and two do not—the shaded loci. MFISys flagged "core" DM mismatches and kept us from reporting them until we resolved the conflicts.

One interpretation of this apparent conflict might be that the two DMs came from different people, a reasonable assumption because the STR profiles are different. The tissue and bone could have coincidently fused when both people died at the same location. Before concluding this, however, we had to examine all of the data carefully. MFISys's display of the STR data is only a representation reported by the laboratory that performed the STR test. The laboratory made its best estimate of what the true STR profile was, based on how it interpreted the raw data, and then reported it to Gene Codes Forensics. Gene Codes Forensics imported the data into MFISys. It wasn't long before we realized that the original raw data had the potential to tell a different story than the one presented in MFISys.

In the table above, two 10 alleles (shaded) are missing from the DM analysis 1 (first line), and a 13 allele is missing from the last locus (far right, shaded) in DM analysis 2. After inspecting the original electropherogram, we found these alleles were present but below the calling parameter programmed into the instrument. Once we knew this, we would have concluded that these two analyses were really not in conflict because the differences were easily explainable by allelic dropout.

Another example was not so easily interpreted.

TABLE 8. SAMPLE MIXUP

DM 10001 1	XX	14/15	19	21	14/15	29/30	13/16	11	11/12	12/13
DM 10001 2	XX	15/16	16/17	21/22	10/13	31.2/32.2	14/19	12/13	10/11	11

Here were STR profiles of two completely different females. DM sample 1 was a tissue sample removed from around the bone by Bode. DM sample 2 was a tissue sample that had been reextracted at the OCME, supposedly from the same sample that had been submitted to Bode. Simply examining the MFISys representation of the data in the table told us that the profiles were from different people. The DMs had the same DM core number, which is why MFISys flagged them. Erik had to resolve the conflict before we could use the DM to make an ID. Erik determined that there was no commingling but that a sample mixup occurred during retesting. Because this mistake was documentable, he crossed out DM sample 1 in MFISys, so that it could never be used to make a match.

We resolved most conflicts by retesting. If resampling of the original DM and subsequent retesting gave the same results as the first testing, we assumed the conflict occurred because of commingling.

For months, Erik worked through the MFISys conflicts. However, not all of them were due solely to allelic dropout, commingling, or sample mixups during retesting. And he was beginning to wonder whether another, more widespread, mechanism might be at work.

The list of possible conflicts grew as Erik began looking at mtDNA and SNPs. Simple mtDNA conflicts existed for various reasons, including miscalling by the Celera autocalling software, mtSAS. This was artificial-intelligence software Celera developed to minimize human intervention in calling mitotypes. Simple STR and mtDNA conflicts were often resolved by examining the original STR electropherograms or mitochondrial sequencing data.

Some of the conflicts were not simple and obviously came from other sources such as commingling, sample mixup, or cross-contamination.

At the same time Erik was looking for more systematic reasons for the conflicts he was seeing, Amy Mundorff had been complaining to me and to the second-floor DNA identification unit about problems she found during her anthropological review of RMs. She was finding that some of the RMs had duplicate parts, such as two right hands. Most disturbing was that the two right hands had the same DNA profiles.

In the middle of September 2003, while working through the MFISys conflicts list, Erik identified a new quality problem. It surfaced when data that should match did not. For example, during STR testing, we usually employed overlapping tests to give us the 13 different regions of the DNA we use to match STR profiles. Two loci in these systems overlapped, which gave us a good feeling when they matched. That is, both STR typings were consistent and, second, the samples had not been mixed up. However, Erik found that sometimes one test gave a complete STR profile but the other gave nothing. Both systems should give at least positive test results.

Then in October 2003 Erik discovered an error in the way robots transferred samples from parent to daughter plates. In tracking down the source of the problem, he noticed that some STR profiles were duplicated on daughter plates from DMs having extra-large amounts of DNA in their extracts.

Duplicate microtiter plates, or daughter plates, were prepared by transferring DNA extracts from parent, or stock, plates to daughter plates using a robotic arm. After transferring the DNA from one set of DMs, the tips used to transfer the liquid on the robotic arm were washed six times. Then the same robotic arm was used to prepare another set of parent-to-daughter plates from a different set of DMs.

The problem occurred after a fixed-tip robotic arm transferred DNA extract from a sample having an abnormally high concentration of DNA. During the preparation of the next set of duplicate plates, a small amount of DNA from the first set was transferred to the second set. Erik noticed that the STR profiles from the first DM set were showing up in the second DM set.

Erik and Elaine came to me with the problem. We reasoned that the problem could not be widespread because a significant number of DMs had no STR profiles. If it had been widespread, we would have been inundated with mixtures. We were not. Second, the problem had originated from only DNA extracts having large amounts of DNA. If the contamination were widespread, we would have expected to find multiple mixtures of STR profiles in most of the DMs.

Early on, Bode recognized the potential for contamination and established a procedure to reanalyze all mixtures. That meant reextracting and reanalyzing all bones that gave STR mixtures. My laboratory instituted a similar policy for tissue samples. It was a conservative approach based on our understanding that inadvertent mixtures were a possibility.

However, simply finding the same STR profile in parent-to-daughter plates did not automatically flag a problem. That is, it did not establish that we had either contamination or a sample mixup. The World Trade Center remains were badly fragmented, so having multiple microtiter plates with the same STR profile was expected. Proving that a problem existed required an in-depth investigation. Sorting out the extent of the problem took months.

The bottom line was that after sorting out the problem, Erik could explain many of the previously unexplainable inconsistencies and some of the duplicate RM remains Amy had found. The overriding concern, of course, was whether we had erroneously returned remains to families. Amy and Katie investigated this and learned that a handful of families had received incorrect DMs inadvertently. All but four of these were small fragments that would not have been expected to yield DNA test results, which confirmed Erik's original premise of how the problem occurred. Several other DMs had not been released and were still at the OCME, and Shiya immediately set them aside so that they could not be released. Amy checked these DMs with an eye toward reanalysis. Four had to be reanalyzed. Three of these gave no test results, again confirming Erik's premise, while the fourth gave the same STR profile as the parent DNA extract, indicating there was no contamination of this sample.

None of the released DMs resulted in a misidentification. The worst that happened was that we had returned additional pieces to a handful of families incorrectly.

As had been our policy from the first day, our actions were guided by our concern for the families. Shiya contacted the affected families in April 2004.

28 OUT OF THE BOX

Through August 2002 and into the middle of 2003, identifications dwindled markedly. A small upsurge in June 2003 buoyed my spirits—we had 13 new ones—but I was far from satisfied. Based on some of the identifications we made over the past year, when we combined metadata and DNA typing, I felt we could do better. I was looking for novel approaches. I did realize that any approach rested on how quickly Gene Codes Forensics programmed new functionality into MFISys.

Out-of-the-box thinking always carries risks and, by definition, likely failure. In my mind, if a novel approach resulted in only one new identification, it had not failed, regardless of the time and expense. I was willing to risk failure and severe criticism from my colleagues and staff.

In an e-mail addressed to me, Charles Brenner discussed SNPs. He had presented his views at the KADAP meeting in early July. He estimated, based on the SNP data he had been analyzing, that we had another 200 new identifications sitting in the pipeline. After reading the e-mail, I had to smile. It was typical Charles. He had become a specialist in dangling enticing morsels to buoy my hopes since almost the beginning. Unfortunately, his ambitious predictions rarely met his own expectations. I did not care. It was always heartening to know that there might be additional identifications lurking in the weeds somewhere.

Since my meeting with David Feldt in September 2001, I believed that metadata might become important. I was not entirely sure how to use it in a meaningful way and then combine it with

DNA to tease out more identifications. One such method had its genesis in December 2002 after I read a *USA Today* article while I was visiting my daughter in Washington State. At the time, I called Ralph Ristenbatt, asked him to find the article, and then requested that he initiate a study into how the buildings fell. I thought it might be possible to locate people within the rubble based on where they worked. Ralph expressed his doubts but dove into the project. He learned that the New York City Fire Department had been collecting grid locations of the remains. He contacted the *USA Today* reporter and obtained his data files. It sounded promising, but at the time there was not much STR data in MFISys linked to grid locations. Another problem was that the FDNY did not begin collecting grid data until sometime in October 2001, after thousands of the remains had been recovered.

The second time the idea surfaced was when Katie Sullivan and I were with a number of firefighters in spring 2003. We had been invited to give a World Trade Center update to firefighters at their center in Lower Manhattan, my second meeting with firefighters there. The first time, I gave a formal lecture about the scope of the World Trade Center DNA effort and the current status of the DNA identification process. This meeting was more informal. The fire department served lunch, and Katie and I indulged, though answering questions between bites of chicken Parmesan. Near the end of the session, one firefighter mentioned that the department had data that might pinpoint which firefighters should have been together when the buildings fell.

The germ of the idea I had tucked away in December suddenly made sense. I remembered Ralph's work and the information he had obtained from the *USA Today* reporter. I remembered that the World Trade Center site had been divided into a two-dimensional, checkerboard grid—an important fact. Each recovered human remain had been assigned a grid number. Or I thought they had.

Neither the remains recovered prior to early October 2001 nor those taken to Staten Island had grid numbers—the latter had a notation indicating that they had been from the landfill—but that did not matter. The checkerboard divided the World Trade Center site across the north and south ends, A to Z, and from 1 to 21 along the east and west sides. Each square of the checkerboard was 75 x 75 feet and had a numeric designation, such as O15 or E06.

FIGURE 4. WORLD TRADE CENTER GRID

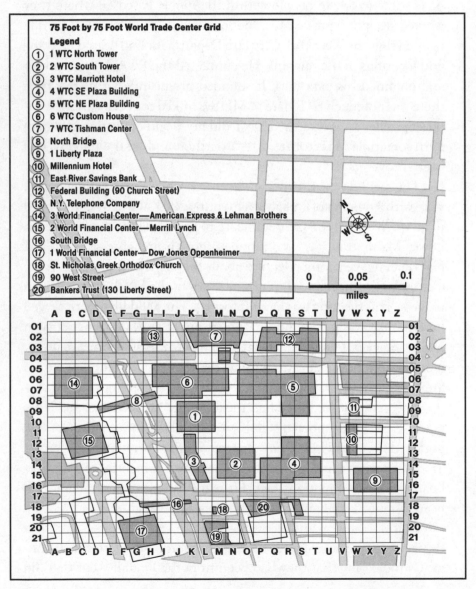

75 Foot by 75 Foot World Trade Center Grid
Legend
① 1 WTC North Tower
② 2 WTC South Tower
③ 3 WTC Marriott Hotel
④ 4 WTC SE Plaza Building
⑤ 5 WTC NE Plaza Building
⑥ 6 WTC Custom House
⑦ 7 WTC Tishman Center
⑧ North Bridge
⑨ 1 Liberty Plaza
⑩ Millennium Hotel
⑪ East River Savings Bank
⑫ Federal Building (90 Church Street)
⑬ N.Y. Telephone Company
⑭ 3 World Financial Center—American Express & Lehman Brothers
⑮ 2 World Financial Center—Merrill Lynch
⑯ South Bridge
⑰ 1 World Financial Center—Dow Jones Oppenheimer
⑱ St. Nicholas Greek Orthodox Church
⑲ 90 West Street
⑳ Bankers Trust (130 Liberty Street)

0   0.05   0.1
miles

If firefighters really had been dispatched in groups, which the fire-fighters had said, it meant that they probably had died together. So if one firefighter in a dispatched group had been identified, the remains of the others should be in the same approximate location, hopefully within the same grid. It sounded like something I could work with.

There were caveats, of course. Everything with the World Trade Center work had caveats, it seemed. An important one concerned the distribution of remains in the grid. Were they distributed in a normal pattern? That is, were the remains spread out evenly? Could we reliably predict how spread out the remains from a single person might be? If we couldn't, this would be another idea without merit.

The recovery process had been anything but precise, and anyone who had watched it on TV knew this. Later, John Cartier, who had been a part of the rescue-recovery effort, and Amy Mundorff, who spent a lot of time at the World Trade Center site, explained how the bulldozers and cranes, their huge grapplers pulling, tugging, and pushing, had moved the rubble around. They were concerned that this process had spread the remains enough to make grid studies useless. It had to be a consideration. But without checking, we would never know. And even if the grapplers had shoved the remains around, the extent was unknown. I believed the remains would likely be located reasonably close to the building where people had worked and died.

How quickly and easily could I get the information to test the hypothesis?

First, I needed the list of firefighters who had been dispatched in groups, and I also wanted a list of every non–member of service who died, where they had worked, and on which floor and in which tower they were most likely located when the buildings fell. I also wanted a list of all the DMs and their grid locations. It took more than a month to get the information. However, when I received the firefighter information, I learned that the information was not precisely what the firefighters had said. True, many of the missing firefighters had "group" designations, but a high percentage did not.

After a couple of weeks, Raju handed me the grid location of the

DMs, a copy of which I gave to Mike Hennessey, who forwarded it to Howard Cash so that he could put it into MFISys. I knew it would take time before the data would be in MFISys, so I started working through a three-inch-thick printout in a three-ring binder of DMs and their grid information. I learned that I could trace the remains of a single person, often in a single grid. Also, there seemed to be clear distribution of the remains. How large? I could not tell because there was too much data to sort through it manually.

My first foray into the data was encouraging.

I also discovered that the DMs from a single person seemed to be more or less in sequential order. This, too, was encouraging, although only approximately 30 percent of the DMs had a grid number, which was unfortunate. I hoped that would not necessarily derail what I was trying to accomplish. This was in early May. My heart attack delayed the work until June.

After returning to work in June, I realized that examining the data grid by grid would take months or longer. The project was intriguing, but I wanted to get a feel for whether the project was worth Gene Codes Forensics's time and effort.

I chose one grid, L09, to use as a pilot project. The grid contained only 36 DMs, which means that only 36 pieces had been removed from this grid during recovery. Such a small number meant I could do the work manually and hopefully learn something I could use later. Also, L09 had no suspected firefighters, which was important, too, because our mission was to identify all the remains, not only members of the service or civilians.

Thirteen of the 36 remains had been identified. From MFISys, I learned that 11 had no STR profiles, which meant I would have to rely on mtDNA and/or SNP typing. That would have to wait for some future time. The remaining 12 DMs had partial STR profiles, none of which had a sufficient number of loci to make an identification. This is what I expected. Examining the partial STR profiles showed that two DMs appeared to have come from two of the thirteen identified people. The STRs of four other DMs were sufficiently different to show that they were from missing people who had yet to be identified. Maybe I was on to something. The work was tedious and time consuming, yet I thought the effort might bear fruit. After looking at the hard copy of the grid printout and from studying grid L09, I had little doubt that I could identify additional pieces from previously identified people. However, new identifications mattered the most. I reasoned that, if there were pieces-to-pieces matches, new identifications might be there too.

I looked up the names of those identified in L09 and found where they worked. It was an interesting revelation. Each worked in the North Tower, World Trade Center 1. That was good because L09 was in the World Trade Center 1 footprint (see Figure 4). They worked anywhere from the 85th to the 110th floors. I wondered whether this meant that I was looking at people who had been from a strata of floors that had compacted on top of each other, or were they moving inside the building in a group when they died? Perhaps both. These questions might never be answered. According to James Glanz and Eric Lipton in their book *City in the Sky*, no one above the 104th floor made it out.

After learning where each of the thirteen identified people worked, I discovered something else: two worked for the same company on the 85th floor, two worked for a different company on the 101st floor, and two worked for a third company on the 92nd floor. I couldn't help but speculate that those who worked on the same floor and worked for the same company must have known each other. I had three pairs of people whom I thought might have known each other; maybe they had been friends.

Then I thought, suppose only one person in each of these pairs had been identified? What were the chances I could identify the other simply by comparing the DNA typing from the personal effects or running kinship analyses against the unidentified DMs found inside this grid? It was an enticing thought that would have to wait until MFISys had the proper functionality.

Once MFISys had the grid locations of the DMs, I located the other grids where the pieces of those 13 people identified in grid L09 had been found. Then, using a spreadsheet, I made a scatter plot with L09 forming the central grid.

The graphic below illustrates what I found.

The graphic is a copy of the original spreadsheet I used for my L09 grid studies. The light gray squares represent a spread of 4 grids in each direction away from L09. Each dark-shaded square represents where the additional remains of someone identified in L09 had been found. Each different shade represents the remains of a single person. For example, the six shaded squares containing the number 1 show that the remains of this person were spread in six different grids, as well as in L09. The darker shaded square containing the number 2 shows that this person was found in two grids in addition to L09.

FIGURE 5.   SPREAD PATTERN OF REMAINS RECOVERED IN GRID L09

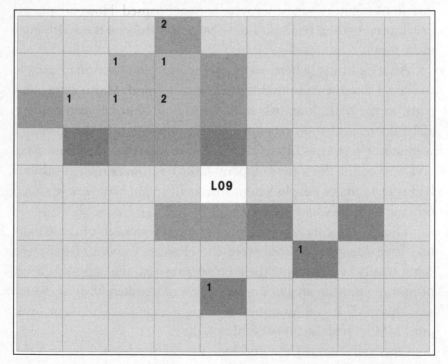

With few exceptions, the majority of the pieces from each person came from within a four-grid radius of the central grid, L09. Clearly, the recovery process and how the buildings fell had imposed a distribution of the remains. However, the majority of the remains had been distributed more or less predictably. Additionally, the grid spread fell within the North Tower's footprint.

If two of the victims, friends, and/or coworkers had been together when the buildings fell, and I knew the grid where one of them had been found, and if there had been STRs, SNPs, or mtDNA typing from their remains, I believed I had a fighting chance to pinpoint the remains of the friend, if they had been recovered. Initially, I thought the method seemed equally applicable to civilians and firefighters.

In truth, the method might be easier to apply to firefighters because several of them were known to have been together. I asked Raju for an electronic file of all those who died and their work locations. I originally thought I might have to contact the families to find out who was with whom when the buildings collapsed. However, simply knowing which floor the people were on and the company for which they worked might suffice.

These data led me to another pilot project.

This time I chose a company instead of a grid, Marsh & McLennan, located on the 93rd to 100th floors of the North Tower, Tower 1. I looked up which Marsh employees had been identified at this time in June 2003 and prepared a scatter plot in a spreadsheet showing the grids where their DMs had been found. A portion of the spreadsheet is shown in Figure 6.

The grid coordinates are shown on the left and across the top. The graphic displays only a fraction of the entire World Trade Center site, which went from A to Z and from 1 to 21. The footprints of the Twin Towers are outlined in black, with the North Tower near the center of the diagram and the South Tower on the lower right. Each asterisk inside the grids represents an identified remain from someone who worked at Marsh. The graphic is a rectangle because I was working with a spreadsheet.

Interestingly, greater than 80 percent of the identifications remains were found within the footprint of the North Tower—exactly where they should have been. Also apparent was that the remains from a single person were spread out, which is what I found in grid L09.

Next, I wanted to compare the STR profiles of the personal effects of the missing in Marsh & McLennan and compare them to the STR profiles of the unidentified DMs. I realized that any matches I might find would be tentative. In fact, I expected that most, if not all, would have partial STR profiles and multiple instances of allelic dropout. Proving any of these identifications would require a lot of additional work. Still, I hoped this data might point me toward new identifications.

I prepared a spreadsheet containing STR profiles from the personal effects and looked only for direct matches. Then I sorted them against the STR profiles of the DMs from the grid. The reality of the data hit me hard. Nothing exploded off the spreadsheet screaming, "You found me!"

I did locate one barely marginal match, which would have required proving allelic dropout in both the DM and the personal effect for it to pan out. Still, it was better than nothing. However, while the match was not impossible, making the identification stick would have to wait for mtDNA or SNPs or both. It was a lot to ask. In the end, I felt my work showed that the grid studies held promise.

The pilot projects were tedious. I had already consumed two weeks and two weekends, and I had barely scratched the surface. Also, my other work was suffering. I needed software help. I talked to Tracy Beeson of Gene Codes Forensics and asked if she would program my grid approach into MFISys.

The following Wednesday, I presented the result of my grid work to the families at our regularly scheduled family meeting. Howard Cash showed up unexpectedly, of course, and was taking notes. The next time I saw him, he handed me a printout prepared by Tracy. Although their results were somewhat sobering, they confirmed what I

FIGURE 6. PATTERN OF MARSH & McLENNAN EMPLOYEES
REMAINS RECOVERED

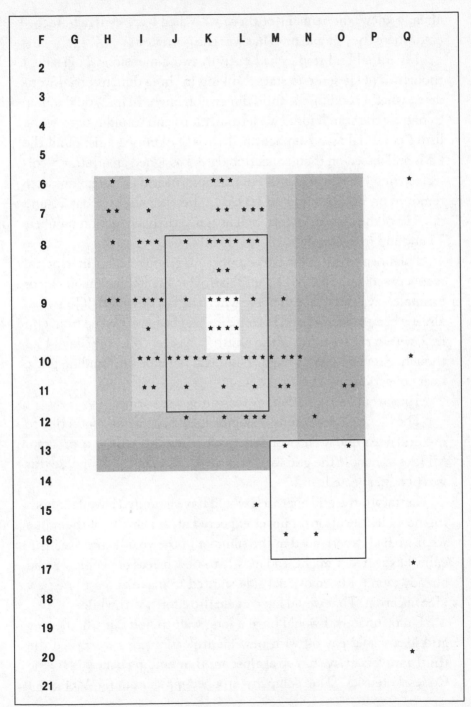

already knew: the remains of those who died were generally recovered where they should be. That was the good news.

My initial grid studies had been in two dimensions. Logically, I thought it made sense to start thinking in three dimensions. I wondered whether adding the third dimension might help. Would it help to narrow the search for new identifications and would it narrow the list of potential as-yet-unidentified DMs? I obtained a list of all the DMs and, based on their collection date, I assigned an arbitrary "collection number" to each date. For example, in grid G09, remains were removed on 12/13/01 and on 1/31/02. These represented day 75 and day 113 of the recovery effort. So I assigned them collection numbers 75 and 113 respectively.

I planned to use collection numbers to group remains in a logical recovery sequence so that I could narrow my search parameters. For example, say John was with Steve when the buildings fell. If John had already been identified and his remains had been recovered from grid L09, within the footprint of the North Tower on collection day 113, I thought Steve's remains might be in the same or surrounding grids, near collection day 113.

Time would tell whether my reasoning was correct.

The Gene Codes Forensics engineers did not wholly subscribe to my grid idea and were wondering whether the effort to program MFISys to handle the grid work was worth their effort. I suppose this was not unexpected.

Certainly, the grid approach would have a limited payoff for finding new identifications. I never expected an avalanche of them like what we had experienced in the summer of the year before. Realistically, I expected it might lead mostly to new pieces of people we had already found. My emotional side wanted to make at least one new identification. That would have made the effort worthwhile.

Unfortunately, I would have a long wait to find out whether my grid idea would pay off with new identifications. As we passed the third anniversary, we ran up against another funding issue with Gene Codes Forensics. The company stopped programming MFISys. I began thinking that this phase of the work would have to be pushed off into the "new technology" phase of the work.

Erin Ryan was a young anthropologist who was teaching science in California before joining the World Trade Center effort in April 2003. She had been Amy Mundorff's roommate when they were students at Syracuse University. So when she left her job in California and grabbed the opportunity to come east to help Amy, it was a good decision for us and the World Trade Center work.

Erin thought that checking the medical examiners' records in the database for pieces that logically fit with existing ones might help to reassociate pieces from an already identified person. I thought it was a good idea. For example, she found a torso with a ripped blue shirt that she thought might link to a lower arm having a fragment of blue shirt attached. Again, it was a lot of work for a low payoff, but most out-of-the-box thinking at that stage of the World Trade Center investigation had a low payoff. She brought these cases to me, and I checked the STR profiles to see if there were matches. We were successful in one instance and others seemed promising.

Another approach came from Steve Sherry at the National Center for Biological Informatics.

We had a huge number of DMs having partial STR profiles that could not be used to make identifications. In addition, most of these suffered from extensive allelic dropout, so comparing them to a personal effect or doing kinship analysis was next to impossible. Elaine, Noelle, and Erik had been making identifications by reanalyzing the STR electropherograms. They often found an allele that had not been displayed in MFISys that allowed them to make a match. Unfortunately, doing this work manually was a hit-or-miss process. I believed we needed a systematic way to identify allelic dropout and then compare the results to personal effects. The only way to do it efficiently so that we had a chance to find all the relevant STR profiles with allelic dropout was to examine the data electronically.

I spoke to Steve Sherry about the problem. He suggested writing a program to accomplish this; I gave him the go-ahead in July 2003. Steve Niezgoda and Mandy Sozer planned to work with him. Although it would take years to write the program and then have it tested thoroughly against World Trade Center data, I felt it was worth the effort and the delay.

I thought the approach would work because that was precisely what Noelle Umback had been doing manually for months. She had been working through a list of potential identifications, where partial STR profiles were expected. To be successful, Steve Sherry's program had to examine the electronic data from the instruments that produced the electropherograms and then look for STRs that were just poking their heads above the instrument noise.

We learned that a negative was not necessarily a true negative and that usable DNA data might be available for reinterpretation. After examining the original electropherogram, Noelle, Elaine, Erik, and Anca Nicholson often found data that was not reported by the contract laboratory and that was also absent in MFISys. This often led to new identifications.

As we moved into March 2004, it was clear that I needed to move forward with Steve Sherry's project. Steve continued working from his end, but I wanted data faster. If I was going to complete the DNA work in September 2004—my artificial deadline—I needed to move this phase of the project along.

Through Mecki Prinz, I contacted Dr. Mark Perlin, the founder of Cybergenetics Corp, a Pittsburgh corporation that was marketing an artificial-intelligence DNA program, True Allele, that could find and identify alleles in electropherograms. True Allele is a robust commercial product that had been used in a number of laboratories throughout the world, including the Forensic Science Services in Great Britain. Barry Duceman had validated it for his DNA databasing laboratory at the New York State Police Department in Albany.

Mecki, Elaine, Erik, and I met with Mark on April 6 to discuss the logistics of using True Allele to reanalyze the MFISys database of STR profiles. Mark agreed with me that this was doable.

I contacted Tom Brondolo about the contractual process. I feared that this contract would go the way of the Gene Codes Forensics contract. I did not want another stop-and-start situation. Catherine DeNiro, the OCME contracts officer, worked with Mark to set up a contract. This was going smoothly, much more so than I could ever remember with other contracts. Something had to give. It was the city way.

In May, Elaine and I were discussing True Allele and how I thought it should be used to analyze the World Trade Center data. I asked, "Do you think I'm nuts for doing this?" Without looking up from her notepad—maybe she just didn't want to look me in the eye—she hesitated a moment before saying "Yes." I was surprised and a bit taken aback and immediately felt I had to justify my position, saying, "I wanted a better way to look at those profiles, something that's not so ad hoc." Then she said, "More systematic—we've already done more than anyone else would have done. But if we get a new identification from it . . ."

Elaine is soft-spoken and sometimes her voice trails off. So if she finished the sentence, I did not hear it. She was less than enthusiastic about the project, but she was not about to let a chance to identify more of the missing slip by without giving it a chance.

As the weeks rolled into late summer 2004, my September 30 deadline was creating angst, which, even without the pressure of making identifications, was taking its toll on my staff.

By August, Elaine's group was averaging between 240 and 260 piece-to-piece reports monthly. After some research, Elaine said that her group would have to report approximately 2,500 piece-to-piece matches to meet my deadline. It was impossible. At their current rate, it would have taken nearly ten months. Most of these matches, however, would be tough because they included partial profiles. Many also had SNP and/or mito conflicts that Erik would have to sort out first. Erik was pulling his hair out working through the existing QC conflicts and did not need an additional burden. Elaine had been working doggedly to pull the data together so that we could track them. In all, there was more work than there were days left.

Elaine came to me for help. As she explained the problem, I realized that my September 30 deadline was unrealistic and I had to compromise or extend the project almost indefinitely. A deadline was important, but it did not have to be *this* specific deadline. My overriding concern was that I wanted this group out from under this project.

I asked her, "How many of the twenty-five hundred are simple matches without conflicts?" I meant, how many of the piece-to-piece matches did not require extensive work beyond simply reporting them out.

She thought for a moment. "Maybe five hundred."

We could report out five hundred piece-to-piece matches in two months. It would be close, but well within reach. We agreed on new guidelines: Elaine would concentrate on reporting new identifications, matches that met stats but did not have conflicts. She would consider conflicts only if they involved larger pieces. She would shift problem DMs, those that might never reveal an identification, into the "new technology" phase, and whoever headed the project at that point would concentrate on them. Many of these had major problems that might never be solved.

I still aimed for the September 30 deadline for reporting out new identifications and the easy piece-to-piece matches. After September 30, I planned to spend the remainder of the year getting the DNA and identification data and other records in order so that someone else could take over. The families needed a stop date, a pause date, as Chuck Hirsch liked to call it. And so did we.

On August 31 Elaine was in my office. We had been discussing our individual futures when she said something I had been waiting to hear. Before that day, I could only guess when it would come. She said, "I don't think we have any more new identifications."

It was an incredible moment. Those few words sent an immediate shock surging through me. I felt both giddy and incredibly sad. A year earlier, while Steve Niezgoda was still working with us, I had said to him that if we had two consecutive months without identifications, I thought we would be finished. I had never shared this with anyone else. In the weeks before then, I had been thinking that when the pipeline went dry, we'd be finished. That's exactly what Elaine was telling me: the pipeline had run dry. Nearly three years after the attacks, there was a light at the end of the tunnel.

The September 30 deadline came and went. Elaine and I had another conversation about deadlines. She had identified additional DMs that had to go to Bode, work that would not be completed until February 2005. Still, the work was winding down. She set up a schedule so that most of her World Trade Center staff could return to the casework DNA laboratory by January. She and Erik would continue working until March 2005.

PART III

WINDING DOWN AND MOVING ON

29 IDENTIFICATIONS: THE THIRD YEAR

	MISSING IDENTIFIED	DNA IDENTIFICATIONS	REMAINS IDENTIFIED
April 30, 2003	1,166	776	5,942
April 30, 2004	1,552	812	8,448

The statistics show how frustratingly slow it was finding and documenting the 36 new identifications we found in the third year after September 11. New identifications were few and far apart, but the work never ceased. Elaine Mar and her group doggedly plowed through DNA and metadata. Erik Bieschke continued to focus on quality issues. Mike Hennessey pumped out admin reviews. Kecia Harris, Jen Simon, Anca Nicholson, and Michele Martinez stayed busy matching DNA profiles, Anca and Michele reporting them. It took the entire year, but through their efforts, we also managed to repatriate 2,506 pieces.

In April 2004, Elaine approached me with a possible new identification. It had been in the works but had lingered, unfortunately, because the kinship statistics did not meet the KADAP barrier. We had a toothbrush that matched one of the victim samples, and although its DNA profile had sufficient statistics, we could not prove who brought the toothbrush to the Family Assistance Center. For us, it meant a break in the chain of custody, which kept us from making the identification. Katie Sullivan spoke to the husband of the missing woman in early 2003 and asked for another sample. She also sent him a DNA collection kit. He never returned it.

Elaine thought someone should call the family. I wanted the identification just as badly and agreed to make the call. To make the identification, we needed a toothbrush from his daughter. Without it, the identification would be impossible and the remains would never be returned to the family. It was a haunting thought.

Whenever I had to call a family, I preferred to be alone. I needed time to gather my thoughts and formulate what I wanted to say. Normally, I would shut the door to my office so that no one would disturb me. At this point in the investigation, it was more than just calling a family to ask for a sample. How do you call nearly three years after the fact? How do you call to say "We might have found your wife, but without your help, we cannot prove it"? As the phone rang, I tried to stay calm. A man answered, and I asked to speak to the husband. He acknowledged who he was, and then I introduced myself. I explained who I was and provided a brief overview of our World Trade Center DNA work.

Then I said, "Sir, I'm afraid I need your help."

He was curious and, I suspect, a bit confused. "How can I help you?" he asked.

"I apologize for calling like this, sir, but I believe we have found your wife. Unfortunately, I need your help to prove it," I said, praying he was not angry about my dropping such a bombshell out of the clear blue.

This was an unusual call, my first explicitly mentioning a pending identification. These calls were typically more generic, and we purposely omitted or minimized the details. So while I felt confident we had found his wife, telling him anything about a possible identification went against our policy to date. It was also an extraordinary circumstance because nothing would be certain or finalized until we had the toothbrush, had completed the DNA testing, and then matched that to the DM. What if the DNA testing failed? What if it wasn't his wife? I would have raised his expectations only to dash them with a future phone call.

I heard nothing for several very long seconds. I guessed he was trying to get a grip on what he had heard. Finally, my nervousness compelled me to say something, and I said, "I realize this is a shock, but—"

"It's okay, you are just doing your job," he interrupted.

My mind was saying, Actually, this is really an obsession, not just my job. Instead, I said, "I need a DNA sample from your daughter and also from you so that I can prove that we have really found your wife."

We talked a little about the type of sample I needed and why. I also explained why we could not make the identification with the information we had. He hesitated. I offered to come to him and collect the samples personally. I did not want to risk sending a kit and then having him not return it.

Again, silence prevailed. Finally he said, "Can you call me tomorrow?"

He wanted time to think. I had no choice but to agree, although the thought that he was putting me off sped through my mind. He explained how concerned he was for his daughter. Apparently she had trouble adjusting to the September 11 events, and he was nervous about broaching the subject with her. I agreed and we hung up. I sat motionless for a minute or two thinking about what a shock my call must have been for him. Still, he had been gracious.

The next day he called and said he preferred to collect the samples himself. Then he said, "I don't want to meet you." That took me aback. I expect it would have been painful and having me there might have resurrected those terrible memories. He also did not want his daughter to know about our conversation. Over the next few minutes, I explained how to collect the samples and package them. He took my home address and we hung up. The samples came about a week later. I gave them to Elaine, who instituted the testing process. We made the official identification a couple of weeks later.

May 2004 brought a flurry of new identifications because we were using all the information at our fingertips. In an e-mail, Elaine wrote that more families were donating reference samples, such as toothbrushes, and these led to new identifications. Mike Hennessey found that many of the missing people had invalid exemplars. New ones were being pulled and tested, which gave new data. New information from families or medicolegal investigators allowed Mike to sort many of the problem admin reviews. There were data that had never been put into MFISys, reanalysis of DMs using new techniques provided additional DNA data, and Erik continued solving conflicts that led to new identifications.

I prayed this trend would continue. I knew it would not.

30 THE TERRORISTS

When the planes crashed into the Twin Towers, and we began receiving remains, I never seriously thought we would ever recover the remains of the terrorists. I believed the crash and subsequent explosion had blasted them into tiny bits and pieces, most of which had probably vaporized in the ensuing fireball. Although I hoped differently, I believed the passengers on the planes suffered a similar fate.

The reality and surprise was that we had identified many of the passengers. Rumor had it that the terrorists had herded the passengers into the back of the planes. If that was true, it could explain why we were finding their remains. Perhaps the crash and subsequent explosion fragmented them and blew them away from the fireball. However it happened, it was a blessing for the families.

At many of our family meetings and also in private conversations with family members, I fielded questions about the terrorists' remains. Their concern, of course, was and probably still is that their loved ones' unidentified remains and the terrorists' unidentified remains are forever commingled. None of us wants this. Even thinking that these innocent people must rest forever with these murderers is infuriating.

These queries often went something like, "Do you think we will ever find the terrorists?"

Initially, I would say, "I doubt it." However, doubting and knowing were different things. Before we could separate the terrorists' and the victims' remains, we needed examples of the terrorists' DNA.

In spring 2002, Chuck Hirsch and I discussed trying to obtain DNA profiles of the terrorists. We reasoned that the FBI might have either the terrorists' DNA or their STR profiles. I doubted the FBI would have mitotypes of the terrorists. It certainly would not have their SNP types. By once again turning to the FBI for help, we were propelling ourselves into another exasperating bureau experience. A reasonable time frame within which to expect this information should have been a couple of weeks, maybe a month. Instead, it took longer than a year. If only I could have been a fly on the wall when this topic came up in the FBI's offices. What were they thinking? At one point, I questioned whether they truly empathized with the families. I wanted to believe they did. The delay likely had something to do with some weird and convoluted process relating to national security; I'm sure the DNA profiles of these cowards was felt to pose a national threat. How? I had no clue. Or maybe it was simply bureaucratic crap. To be generous, maybe they had to obtain the samples and also had not done the laboratory work. If that were the case, my preference would have been for them to have sent us the samples. We would have done the work over the weekend.

Eventually, we received a one-page letter from the FBI containing ten coded STR profiles, presumably those of the terrorists. No names, just a K code, which is how the FBI designates "knowns," or specimens it knows the origin of. These Ks had no names. We were certain these were the terrorists' STR profiles, but there was nothing to identify them as such. Of course, we had no direct knowledge of how the FBI obtained the terrorists' DNA.

Elaine entered the STR profiles into MFISys: two immediate identifications! I was stunned. If these were indeed STR profiles of the terrorists, we had identified two of the bastards, which meant their remains had not vaporized in the fireball.

I have thought about those identifications often. Were they the terrorists who were piloting the planes or were they the ones holding the passengers hostage in the rear of the plane? I guessed the latter. I still doubt the pilots have anything remaining to collect or analyze. Likely, they were vaporized along with many of the innocent victims.

At the February 2003 annual meeting of the American Academy of Forensic Sciences in Chicago, I asked Dr. Dwight Adams, director of the FBI laboratory, whether he would arrange for someone to send the DNA extracts from the terrorists. I reasoned that many of their remains might have badly compromised DNA. Dwight agreed and said he would send the samples. As expected, it did not happen overnight, or even soon, but we had them in-house by October 2003.

Each new data dump meant a check in MFISys for a match to a terrorist. It was actually automatic because MFISys stored the terrorists' STR profiles in a separate database, away from the victims' DNA profiles. If there was a match, a tab in the program turned red. We always knew. Mostly, it remained colorless. By the time we paused, it had turned red three times.

By identifying three of the terrorists, we created a problem: their remains were with those they murdered. Chuck Hirsch and I discussed it and agreed the terrorists' remains did not belong with their victims. In fact, we believed they should not be on American soil. Chuck sequestered them from the other remains.

31 NOW IT'S OUR TURN

April 30, 2004

THE PLANES:
WORLD TRADE CENTER AND AA FLIGHT 587

	NO. WHO DIED	NO. IDENTIFIED	NO. IDENTIFIED BY DNA
AA Flight 11 (Tower)	87	52	45
UA Flight 175 (Tower)	60	27	26
AA Flight 587 (Queens)	265	265	96

WORLD TRADE CENTER MFISys STATISTICS

NO. STR PROFILES	NO. MITOTYPES	NO. SNP PROFILES
52,528	31,155	10,799

In September 2003, Shiya and I took Amtrak's Acela Express from New York to Boston to meet with several of the September 11 families, most of whom lost loved ones who had been on either AA Flight 11, which crashed into the North Tower, or UA Flight 175, which crashed into the South Tower. Along with an NYPD property clerk representative, we gave an overview of our work. We each spoke for approximately forty-five minutes and then offered the families an opportunity to ask questions. Mostly, the questions showed their concern over whether we had sufficient information to make an identification if we found their loved one.

After speaking we set up onstage to welcome family members who had questions. I booted up my laptop with MFISys onboard while several family members formed a queue in front of me, waiting anxiously. One by one they gave me their loved one's RM number, which I entered into MFISys. As I waited for the program to search the World Trade Center database, I found myself studying them carefully. I could not help but notice the apprehension on their faces, a nervous shifting from side to side, an expectant look.

I suppose they were hoping not to hear something like, "I'm sorry, but we need another sample because we can't make the identification yet." During my presentation, I warned that this might be a possibility. Or, I might say, "We have sufficient DNA to make the identification when we find her." Maybe, even, a couple of them were hoping to hear, "I have good news. We just identified him this morning."

I had a surprise, actually two. After entering one RM number into MFISys, I checked the STR profiles. I couldn't believe what I was seeing. We had an identification! It was absolutely clear and unquestionable. MFISys had been programmed to insert a red I into a column next to the DM number that had been reported to the medicolegal investigators. There it was, as clear as could be. I completely lost my cool. "Haven't you been notified?" I blurted to the victim's relative.

He looked at me skeptically. "No," he said.

"Are you sure?" I asked. Now I was getting nervous. I could feel the perspiration building on my head. I had revealed information inadvertently and leaped into uncharted territory.

"Uh, yes." His curiosity was growing. "Is there something wrong?"

"Oh, no. Not at all." I was suddenly at a loss for words. "It's just that—" I motioned to Shiya, who came over and stood behind me. I pointed to the perfectly clear identification. We exchanged a quick glance, acknowledging we had to tell this man something. Who knows what the man was thinking, but he watched anxiously while Shiya and I conferred privately. Shiya pulled him aside and told him what had happened, promising to look up the information when we returned to New York. It was a sweaty-palms moment for me.

Thankfully, there was a logical explanation for what appeared to be a monumental foul-up. MFISys normally highlighted when a DM had been reported to the medicolegal investigators by placing a red I next to the STR profile after the second-floor DNA identification unit reported the identification to the medicolegal investigators. From that point, Amy conducted an anthropological review, and the medicolegal investigators notified the New York City Police Department, and they notified the family. The red I in MFISys was visible only to the DNA staff before the process had had a chance to run its course. I should have immediately realized this when the red I popped up in MFISys.

What are the odds it would happen a second time?

This time it was a brand-spanking-new identification. The second-floor DNA identification unit had not yet found it. Once again, I felt the adrenaline coursing through my body. This time, however, I kept my cool. I calmly explained, "We have enough DNA to make the identification, if we recover your husband." As I spoke, I looked directly at the woman. Tears formed quickly. I suppose she was hoping for more than that. She had been waiting patiently for two years for a word from New York. At that moment, I was New York. New York had come to her and he was sitting in front of her unable to tell her what she needed to know, although New York could have said what she wanted to hear. It would have been the truth. It was all I could do to keep from crying. I wanted to tell her so badly it hurt. When she walked away, I motioned to Shiya, who looked at MFISys, nodded, and then wrote the RM number on a sheet of paper. He would check it out when we returned to the OCME.

Another widow who had toured my laboratory earlier in the year did not approach the stage, but I remembered her, and I noticed she was still wearing her wedding ring. We had recovered her husband's remains in October 2001.

Three weeks after the Boston trip that woman and several other Boston World Trade Center widows came to New York. We met in the first-floor OCME conference room. She was no longer wearing her wedding ring and seemed more relaxed and smiled more easily. I thought maybe she had finally begun to reconcile with her loss and was finally ready to move on with her life. I had seen the opposite too frequently.

In late January 2004 I met with a firefighter's wife in my laboratory. She was upset because we had identified most of the firefighters whom she had been led to believe had been with her husband when the buildings fell, but not him. Naturally, I felt awful. Situations like this happened often. We identified someone who was supposed to be with someone, but not the person who died with them. On the surface it seemed inexplicable. How could we identify only one of two people who died together, especially when we had seen so much commingling of the remains? The answer is both elusive and disturbing. We could explain how the buildings fell and the inaccuracy of the recovery effort. Maybe both people were not really together after the planes hit and before the buildings fell or got separated as they searched for a way out. It often seemed to defy logic. Still, recorded cell phone calls indicated that people were together.

Once again, I turned to MFISys and searched the database using a low sorting stringency for comparing STR profiles. I hoped to find a partial STR profile that might line up with her husband's personal effect.

Nothing.

I wondered whether searching a grid might give me an investigative lead. This was something I rarely did because it took so much time. She handed me a list of seven firefighters who had been in her husband's engine company and supposedly had died with him. I looked up their RM numbers, found the ones who had been identified, and then checked the grids where their remains had been found. Unfortunately, only two of the seven had grid numbers. It was not a lot of information, but it was better than nothing.

One DM popped out at me, what I thought might be a remote possibility. I forwarded the information to Noelle Umback, who examined the original electropherograms. Unfortunately, there was no match; the DM was a piece from a firefighter whom we had already identified.

I felt bad that I did not have reassuring news for her. I was telling her this when I noticed she was still wearing her wedding ring. I commented on it. Tears immediately sprang into her eyes, and she said, "Until I have him back, I will always feel like I'm still married to him."

The comment stunned me, and it took a few seconds before I could collect my thoughts. I pointed to my chest and said, "I believe you will always be married to him in your heart."

She stared at me for a seemingly long time during which I chastised myself for saying anything that might have offended her. Had I stupidly encroached on her private emotional hell? I guess I said what was on my mind because my experience was that family members were always willing to share their thoughts and feelings. Finally, she said, "I know, but I have to bury him first."

Each of these women, everyone who lost a loved one, had to wrestle with how to "move on." It's an individual thing, something each family member has to work out for him- or herself. Sometimes people say they have "closure" or are "transitioning." In my opinion, nothing seems adequate. Shiya prefers "transition," as he believes this is what we do. I prefer moving on. It is a process that I have trouble adequately relegating to a single word or phrase. It is an emotion with which we all wrestle after losing a loved one. I am hardly a psychologist, but it seems to me that those who lost loved ones in the World Trade Center attacks carry a special burden, different from those who lose loved ones in other ways. Losing someone is never easy, regardless of how it happens, and it's something we must each work through for ourselves. However, it seems to me that having someone die after a prolonged illness, while their death is tragic as any loss of life is, it is not unexpected, and the grieving process has the opportunity to run its course. Certainly that loved one will be missed, and there will be a void that no one else can fill, but there was time to say good-bye.

When a husband, wife, child, sibling, parent, or close friend dies suddenly, such as after a heart attack or an automobile accident, the death is a shock. In some respects, it must be similar to what happened at the World Trade Center because there is not sufficient time to put affairs in order, say good-bye, or deal with the logic of the passing. However, unlike for the World Trade Center families, there is a body and a proper burial service that allows the grieving process to begin.

Many of those who lost their loved ones on September 11 have nothing more than pictures, films, or memories to remind them of the wonderful moments they enjoyed. Their loved one—whether a firefighter, a police officer, or someone who worked at the World Trade Center—was simply an innocent person who left home that morning and never returned. For slightly less than half of these families, nothing of their loved ones came home. They have no one to bury.

Then there are the families who had remains returned and had the opportunity to bury them in an appropriate ceremony. Most received only a small fragment of their loved one, sometimes something as small as an inch-long piece of bone, nothing resembling a human body. For these families, the identifications required the ultimate faith in our identification process and in the DNA work. And how difficult was it for them to execute a proper burial while a part or most of their loved one was elsewhere? Many of these families may never experience closure, move on, or transition, and their grieving may well be prolonged, perhaps lasting forever. I completely understand why many families consider the World Trade Center site sacred ground.

Watching and listening to these wonderful people has affected me, too. I had to learn to move on, which I finally realized meant I would never be the same person I was before September 11. Sometimes I wonder whether I will ever be as emotionally stable as I used to be. I certainly do not look at life or people or the world in the same way. I have changed, and the way I approach people is different. I have become more pensive and reserved, no longer the happy-go-lucky, impulsive person I was when I was younger. I am no longer as happy as I once was.

The work had also affected my staff. Elaine Mar often said that she was not sure what she would do once the work was finished, although she had expressed an interest in supervising our missing-persons group, which is what she does now.

When Elaine dropped by my office to chat on May 4, 2004, I decided to broach the topic of a final date for World Trade Center DNA work, which had been on people's minds for months. Elaine's group knew I wanted to complete the work by the end of September. She had written a rather detailed plan of what she felt needed to be done, although no one really believed we could do it. Even if we finished the DNA work on time, data would need to be analyzed. This meant there would be a trickle of DNA reports being sent to the medico-legal investigators for possible new identifications and piece reassociation, and families would have to be notified. This was unacceptable. The families deserved a firm date. They had to know when they could stop hoping.

At the family meeting a month earlier in April, the topic came up and I hedged, saying something fuzzy, suggesting that the third anniversary would mark the end of the DNA work, or the "pause," as Chuck Hirsch preferred. At her subsequent April staff meeting, Elaine mentioned that the anniversary would be the stop date. Like me, she hedged, saying that there might be an extension.

I countered, "There will not be an extension." I was wrong.

Earlier on May 4, Katie Sullivan had poked her head around my door and said, "When is the last day?"

"What last day?"

"The last day for DNA reports?" she said, laughing. She was taunting me, and I knew it. But it was not a question without intent. Katie wanted to stop, so she had come at the right time because I was ready to commit. I knew we needed an end. The OCME had to send letters to the families alerting them that the current phase of identifications would take a hiatus. It would mark the official World Trade Center end date for DNA reports.

"September 30," I said. "September 30 will be the last day the second-floor DNA identification unit will send out DNA reports." After that date, no more new identifications or piece-to-piece matches would be sent to the medical legal investigators. I had chosen the date from thin air, purposely extending the anniversary date by three weeks.

We had a ton of work yet to do. I spoke with Mike Hennessey. I needed to know whether he could complete the bulk of the admin reviews by the end of September. He replied by saying that he had planned to finish by the beginning of September, with the caveat that there could always be glitches, problem cases, of which there might be as many as one hundred that might never be resolved. There might be fewer, and these would be hopelessly mired in ambiguity. Brian Gestring, the ex-MESATT scientist who almost died at the World Trade Center, had formulated an aggressive plan to resolve these over the next few months. Mike speculated that as many as 10 percent might turn out to be new identifications, if they could somehow resolve the metadata problems.

The remainder of Elaine's staff would be pedal-to-the-metal to get the work done and neatly tie up the loose ends. Erik would resolve the dangling quality-control issues. Anca Nicholson and Michele Martinez would continue reporting identifications and piece reassociations waiting in the pipeline. Jennifer Simon and Kecia Harris would continue reviewing STR, SNP, and mito profiles. Elaine would continue working on the elusive and tough identifications.

Eventually, their work would end. I could not help but wonder how each of us would handle working on other projects. I had been lucky. My responsibilities had changed along the way, but Elaine had been knee deep in the World Trade Center work since 2001. I worried about her.

Daniel Lewin, a former Israeli soldier, had been a successful dot-com businessman. He was also most likely the first to die after the World Trade Center attacks. According to an article in the *Daily News* on July 24, 2004, one of the cowardly hijackers stabbed him in the back when he tried to interfere with the hijacking of American Airlines Flight 11. While he probably died on the plane before it crashed, by a twist of fate he was one of the last we identified, an identification that we did not complete until June 3, 2004. The family was notified after that. His identification exemplified the problems we faced.

The small piece of tissue we eventually identified as coming from him had been recovered in 2002. Orchid performed SNP typing and sent us the data in April 2004. Using DNAView, Elaine's staff performed an SNP kinship analysis and then confirmed the identification by STR typing of the toothbrush.

Changes were happening in the OCME before the World Trade Center DNA work started winding down in the summer of 2004, in spite of the fact that the official mission of the OCME remained the same. The DNA laboratory still struggled to make identifications, Shiya's skeleton crew of medicolegal investigators continued working with families, and Amy Mundorff still repatriated human remains reported by Anca Nicholson. The arduous World Trade Center work continued, as did the agency's time-honored official law enforcement mission to ascertain the cause, mechanism, and manner of suspicious deaths and identify the dead. The office unofficially assumed a more prominent role in mass-fatality planning, preparedness, and response.

Additionally, the face of the OCME management changed. Barbara Butcher was appointed the director of medicolegal investigations, which was once Dave Schomburg's responsibility. This was a change that eventually pushed Shiya into a position working for Tom Brondolo and relieved him of his World Trade Center responsibility. Tom assumed more of a leadership role in the agency, and he and Barbara jointly cultivated an agency interest in weapons of mass destruction (WMDs).

To me, this was a radical change in the agency's thinking and philosophy. Given what the entire OCME staff had gone through for the previous three years, the inclination to assume a leadership role in mass-fatality preparedness seemed like a natural step for an agency concerned mainly with identifying the dead and the why and how of death.

I saw the change differently. My job had not changed. The DNA laboratory still had a casework responsibility, and nothing had changed with respect to the World Trade Center work. While Barbara had little impact on my work—she was in charge of the medico-legal investigators who contacted the families—I did need Tom. As he became more and more involved in mass-fatality and hazmat (hazardous material) work, I found it increasingly difficult to get the things I needed to do my work. The biggest problem came when it was time to extend the Gene Codes Forensics emergency contract.

What bothered me the most was that my ability to get the work done was hampered by a commitment to a project that was taking an important manager away from his job. More important, the agency had made a promise to World Trade Center families, but I thought its newfound interest in mass-disaster management had relegated that mission into a background role while promulgating work that was not the charter mission of the office. This change in agency philosophy steadily relegated the functional aspect of the World Trade Center work to the background, though no one would ever admit it, especially to either the families or the press.

From a DNA laboratory management perspective, the need for large numbers of World Trade Center workers had diminished. When the World Trade Center work wound down, I moved WTC staff back into the laboratory to do routine casework. This was critical for our law enforcement mission as well as for the individuals who had dedicated their lives to the World Trade Center families.

Elaine has been writing standard operating procedures for anyone who takes over the project when new technology arrives. She and Howard Cash are now engaged.

Erik Bieschke thought about returning to graduate school, but after leaving the second-floor ID unit, he joined the laboratory's genetics group and wrote a World Trade Center quality-assurance manual in which he outlined his procedures for finding conflicts in the testing.

Mike Hennessey left the group because the Gene Codes Forensics contract ended. He spent many months in Thailand in the wake of the tsunami, as did Howard Cash.

Noelle Umback left the second-floor ID unit in March 2004 and was supervising regular casework. Although she was no longer making identifications, tears often formed in her eyes when we met in the hall to talk.

Anca Nicholson left the second-floor ID unit in April 2005 and began training to do criminal casework.

Jen Simon left New York, now lives in Seattle, and is engaged.

Michele Martinez left the laboratory and joined a fashion company in midtown.

Kecia Harris is working on cases.

Howard Baum and Marie Samples have resumed their daily responsibilities, and Mecki Prinz was chosen by Chuck Hirsch to be the new director of the laboratory after I retired on July 1, 2005.

I firmly believe all medical examiner's and coroner's offices need a comprehensive plan to handle mass-fatality events. This is especially true for an agency that seems in harm's way and has already handled two of historic proportions. Defining what "preparing" means is the crux of the issue, and it might differ depending on the jurisdiction and the agency's resources. New York's hubris and, perhaps, its wherewithal allows it to handle any disaster itself. Now that the World

Trade Center work was "officially" over, except at the OCME, there would be no changing the attitude of, "We did it once, we can do it again."

A small medical examiner's or coroner's office might logically hand off the work to more experienced federal officials. However, a large metropolitan office, like the OCME, might choose to handle the identification process itself, such as we did for the World Trade Center attacks and for American Airlines Flight 587. Beyond assuming responsibility for identifying the dead and preparing properly for such an event, I do not believe medical examiner's offices should either assume a leadership role in mass-fatality preparedness planning or be first responders.

Still, the September 11 experience offered new opportunities for the OCME. The Iraq war and what was touted by President George W. Bush as a solid weapons of mass destruction (WMD) connection to Saddam Hussein propelled many in New York and individuals at the OCME to prepare for imminent WMD attacks. The thinking was and still is that New York City is a likely target. Unfortunately, in my opinion, WMD planning became an obsession with many in the OCME and this obsession altered the office's path and its politics.

I'm not against preparing for WMD attacks. We are all aware that attacks may become a fact of life. We must also be realistic. Nukes are improbable. I believe we know the terrorists' blueprint for future events: multiple coordinated simultaneous or sequential events using conventional explosives. The train attacks in Madrid and the Underground and bus attacks in London and the resort explosion in Egypt underscore this belief. They already have these resources and, for them, it would be easy. Their track record speaks for itself. With the exception of chemical-laced weapons in Iraq and the sarin subway attack in Japan in 1995, there is little evidence showing anything other than chemicals and biologicals as potentially viable WMD candidates.

Does the possibility of a so-called dirty bomb exist? Certainly. Might we see weaponized biologicals and chemicals? Sure. But the conventional explosive route, like the suicide bomber, is their forte. I expect suicide bombers—perhaps with nerve gases or biologicals associated with them—to show up in the United States. Attacks by American radicals like Timothy McVeigh at the Oklahoma City federal building or the vehicular bomb used in the 1993 World Trade Center bombing might escalate, with multiple events occurring simultaneously, perhaps in multiple cities.

The sense I have is that, while terrorism is a distinct possibility, perhaps even imminent, non-terrorist-based mass-fatality events are more likely. Natural disasters are common, and they can be devastating: hurricanes in Florida, earthquakes in California, and tornados in the Midwest kill thousands annually. The 2003 nightclub fire in Rhode Island killed nearly 100 people. The responsibility of the medical examiner is to be prepared to identify those who die as a result of such disasters, including those perpetrated by terrorists.

As we rolled into July 2004, the possibility of another attack loomed. The timing was perfect because the city was gearing up for the Republican National Convention. Terrorist chatter seemed intent on wreaking havoc with the elections, and the intelligence community had been warning of imminent attacks. By the time the RNC began at the end of August, I was becoming more nervous and withdrawn. I hated the thought of having to do it again. Many times I found myself staring into space wondering how I would react. Could I handle it emotionally? I was not sure. Certainly, I was not looking forward to another tour of duty managing another identification effort.

On June 4, 2004, the OCME conducted a tabletop exercise to, as Chuck Hirsch wrote to the OCME staff, "test our ability to respond to a mass-fatality incident in New York City." The idea was to see how well the various OCME departments would work together and respond during the first forty-eight hours after an event. The actual hypothetical event was blind to those of us who participated. The tabletop planners sequenced four simulated attacks: first, a truck rammed a school bus loaded with Jewish children in Lower Manhattan; second, a suicide bomber exploded in a crowd of people watching the *Today Show* live broadcast at Rockefeller Center in Midtown; third, a parked van exploded with two tons of explosives in Midtown not far from the suicide bomber explosion; and fourth, a dirty bomb exploded accidentally in a terrorist's room in a Queens apartment.

The exercise was interesting. After each event in the sequence of escalating events, each department head had to delineate exactly what they would be doing after a certain number of hours. I quickly realized that my DNA laboratory had to be better prepared than it was. We had responded admirably to the largest mass-fatality event in the history of the United States, but we had work to do so that we were not caught flat-footed again. I also realized that how we responded to the World Trade Center attacks might not be appropriate for all mass-fatality events.

I established an in-house committee to study the matter and to formulate a plan. The committee, which I chaired, included Amy Mundorff, Elaine Mar, Lydia DeCastro, Erik Bieschke, Sheila Estacio Dennis, and Mark Desire. I wanted to set up mass-fatality event procedures for the laboratory. We had to review our response to the World Trade Center attacks, ferret out the good from the bad, and then establish procedures for responding if something happened at the Republican National Convention. With barely a month to implement whatever we came up with, this would be our short-term plan, a prelude to a longer-term one for future events.

I also invited Frank DePaolo to sit in on the meetings, as Chuck Hirsch had appointed him the OCME's mass-disaster coordinator. Although each member of the committee, except for Frank, was a member of the DNA laboratory, we each had different responsibilities, suffered different experiences, and had different opinions on how the laboratory had responded to the World Trade Center effort.

Over several weeks, we identified the major World Trade Center problems that we would rather avoid. Our first exercise was to determine the capacity of the laboratory: how many bodies (number of remains) could we handle in-house? That is, how many fatalities, which meant remains plus family samples, did the laboratory have the capacity to analyze? Surprisingly, we did not know, but it was something we had to figure out. This was important because that number would set the parameters for a go-no-go decision with respect to whether we would outsource testing.

I also wanted us to preorganize the laboratory. We had to know who would be responsible for each mass-fatality function: accessioning, extracting, purchasing, STR analysis, identification, and so on. Although DNA testing was our strength, we had to decide which testing regimen to use. Interestingly, we initially decided to use the reverse procedure we commonly use in the laboratory for routine casework. Supplies had been a severe World Trade Center problem. We had to have sufficient supplies to begin processing samples. What if New York City closed down? What would we need to ensure a constant stream of data?

Who would accession, process, and extract the remains? We met with other OCME staff to establish a nomenclature system for remains. The BEAST was not in service and the Integrated System needed an upgrade, so we brought in a software vendor to see whether there might be something available for us to track remains, just a precaution for the Republican National Convention. Staffing the morgue was an issue because of problems that came from our World Trade Center experience. Would the scenario be the same that we used for the World Trade Center? What would our role be in the Family Assistance Centers? Since the Office of Emergency Management would now be in charge, instead of the NYPD, we wanted to exert some influence to ensure we did not have the same problems we had with the World Trade Center. We planned to force ourselves into the Family Assistance Centers. I was adamant about that because the poor work at the Family Assistance Centers created huge problems for my staff.

What about collecting autopsy laboratory samples from remains for DNA testing? This turned out to be another major World Trade Center problem for the DNA laboratory. We wanted a better handle on what samples would be collected and from where. This included a recommendation for better photography of the remains, which would include a photograph of the location from which the ME collected the specimen.

Documentation was also critical. We did not want the shoddy documentation that had been so pervasive for the World Trade Center work and had caused a number of identification problems. We decided that better photography and specimen description were necessary.

Then we tried to tackle how to prioritize which remains would be analyzed first. Obviously, identifying the missing is the first priority, and doing it quickly, albeit correctly, is crucial. There will always be enormous outside pressure to get the work done quickly, at least as far as the public and politicians are concerned.

During the American Airlines Flight 587 work, Chuck Hirsch suggested we analyze the lowest DQ (Disaster Queens) numbers first. Each of the remains from the AA587 crash were given a sequential DQ number. Under the best of circumstances, the lowest numbers should have corresponded to the largest pieces, as these would have been tagged first. It was a good idea that didn't work as well as expected because a fair percentage of the lower DQ numbers did not correspond to the largest pieces. Consequently, we found ourselves analyzing almost all of the remains before making the final identifications. I did not want that to happen again. We obviously had many decisions to make.

32 WHEN IT'S MY TURN

The pressure on the entire OCME staff was tremendous. As the World Trade Center work wound down, I often thought about the people with whom I worked so closely over more than three years. I have fond memories of all of them, even those who made my task difficult. Each had done a damn good job under the most trying of conditions. Many felt the pressure and had to leave the OCME.

One young woman had been working on admin reviews and doing a superb job but could not handle the pressure. Another simply expressed a need to get away. The saddest involved a young woman who felt it most acutely. She had enormous pressure from the World Trade Center work, her personal life, and a select few of her colleagues. One night someone found her hanged from a fence along 30th Street, still clinging to life. Thankfully, she lived. I always thought she was intelligent, dedicated, and engaging—a friend.

I still remember lying in the Key West hospital emergency room in May 2003 with multiple IVs running from my arms, one a morphine drip, the others feeding me whatever the emergency room crew thought I needed. An oxygen mask covered my nose and mouth, and my chest was exploding in unrelenting pain. I kept my eyes shut most of the time, but when I did venture to open them, I always saw a flurry of hyperactivity, human blurs buzzing around me.

I remember hearing a man yell, "What's the pain level now?"

He was talking to me, so I replied exactly as I had for what seemed like an eternity. Same question. Same answer.

"Why isn't he responding? Why isn't he responding?" the same exasperated, anguished voice demanded, words that sent a stark message. I remember whispering into the mask, "I'm going to die." I considered asking, "Am I going to die?" I didn't. Maybe because I really did not want to hear the answer.

Strangely, though, I felt neither frightened nor panicked. Like gravity and the sour taste of lemons, it was a fact: I was going to die. Then a miracle happened. The pain subsided just a smidgen. No question about it. I felt it. A moment later, the doctor yelled yet again from some distance, "How is the pain now?"

He was again asking for a number from zero to ten, with ten being the most intense pain I could ever imagine. I said, "Four." Down from six, which had been my original estimate. Actually, I had no idea what the most intense pain I could imagine might feel like. This was certainly the most intense and prolonged pain I had ever experienced. So I had given a number, probably a starting point from which the physicians could judge how I was doing.

"Thank God," the voice said, calmer now and noticeably relieved.

I was going to live. Spiritual questions abounded. Why had I been spared? Had my mother and father been watching over me? Had one of the World Trade Center victims, perhaps James Cartier, put in a good word for me? Maybe they knew I had more work to do. Who knows? Hopefully, someday, I will learn the truth when it really is my turn.

33 STATISTICS

July 26, 2004: Family Meeting at OCME

Number of Remains: 19,915
Number Identified: 1,560 (5 pending)
Whole Bodies Recovered: 293
Hotline Calls: 14,965
Memorial Park Appointments: 2,301

VICTIMS IDENTIFIED

MODALITY	SINGLE MODALITY: 1,018		MULTIPLE MODALITIES*: 542	
	NO.	PERCENTAGE	NO.	PERCENTAGE
DNA	822	81	472	87
Dental X-ray	98	10	428	79
Fingerprints	52	05	216	40
Photo	11	01	14	03
Remains Viewed	12	01	02	00
Personal Effects	16	02	59	11
Other	07	01	34	06
Body X-ray	03	01		
Tattoos	06	01		

* Multiple modality refers to identifications made where more than one modality was involved, such as DNA and fingerprints.

DEATH CERTIFICATION	NYC DEATH CERTIFICATE BREAKDOWN
Total Reported Missing: 2,749	Judicial Decree (DX) Certificates Only: 1,186
NYC Death Certificates Issued: 2,746	Physical Remains (DM) Certificates Only: 399
Non-NYC Death Certificates Issued: 3	DM Certificate after DX Certificate: 1,161
Total Certificates Issued: 2,746	

On June 2, 2005, Chuck Hirsch read a prepared statement to the Joint Committee on Health and Finance of the Council of the City of New York:

I will begin by providing an update on our World Trade Center operations. After three and a half years of intensive effort, we have identified 1,591 of the 2,749 victims, and have identified 54 percent of the 19,915 recovered remains. Of the identifications made by a single modality, 86 percent have been by DNA, and DNA has been a component in 89 percent of identifications made by more than one modality. Without modern DNA technology, we would have identified only 741 WTC victims; 844 families that now have identifications would have none, and we would have no hope of making additional identifications.

Through the efforts of our personnel and private companies, we have advanced DNA technology to its present limits, and we have virtually exhausted those limits. Consequently, we now have reached the point where additional identifications are unlikely with current technology. This January personnel from our office started telephone notification of next of kin advising them of the pause in new identifi-

cations. These calls have been completed and a follow-up letter has been sent to each of the families. In some instances,
next of kin previously indicated that they do not want any
additional notification or contact, and we are respecting that
choice. Despite this pause in identifications, our WTC identification unit must continue to operate and to serve as a contact point for families.

In July 2005, I had begun my appointment at Pennsylvania State
University and was living temporarily in a university apartment in
State College. At the end of the month I was in New York at the
Slaughtered Lamb in Greenwich Village with several of my ex-
OCME colleagues. I was standing at the bar talking with Elaine and
Anca. Elaine looked at me and said, "We have a new ID."

This was wonderful yet unexpected news. She went on to tell me
that a family had no personal effects but had recently sent swabs from
family members. The DNA laboratory obtained the DNA profiles.
Elaine did the kinship analysis and made the identification. I had
been away from the OCME for almost three weeks and wanted to
know whether there had been other identifications.

"How many IDs do we have?" I asked.

"Fifteen hundred and ninety-six," she said.

I was surprised. It was more than I had expected. Elaine had always wanted to reach the sixteen hundred level, a number we had
discussed several times. On that night we were four shy.

EPILOGUE: DNA MADE THE IDENTIFICATION

We enter life as a child, live life to the fullest, and then exit. How we do this is really up to us. Few of us knowingly follow a set path. We live our lives, sleep in our own beds, and make our own decisions within the framework of the life we choose. We make plans for our futures and set out to accomplish our goals. However, the unknown always lurks there, waiting, and often tosses in the proverbial monkey wrench, seemingly to disrupt those plans, perhaps to see how we will react. Some of us do well and respond appropriately and adapt, some cannot. Sometimes others choose our path for us. That's what happened on September 11. The World Trade Center attacks sent reality crashing down at my feet and thrust me into a situation for which I was ill prepared.

My job description was easy: identify those who perished and return them to their families. This was a scientific effort that turned into an obsession. It was a seemingly simple task that turned complex, an intense source of frustration. It was tedious, difficult, and emotionally draining for me and for my staff. While the science was complex, it was the duration of the still-incomplete project that extracted its toll. The human remains have also proven to be a worthy opponent, and the challenge to find usable DNA in them is ongoing.

In the fall of 2001, I started searching for novel ways to analyze the remains and embraced a myriad of technologies. My goal was to bring loved ones home using whatever reliable technology I could find. This endeavor created numerous problems for me, my staff, and the medicolegal investigators. I also weathered criticism from my forensics colleagues.

I decided early in October 2001 to venture away from the tried and true—the STRs used daily in forensic work worldwide—because I knew in my heart that path would not return enough of the missing to their families. Unfortunately, the path I chose left my staff emotionally drained and created problems for my laboratory's daily routine. My decision dragged out the testing by at least two years, probably longer, and it almost killed me. While I am sorry for the extra work and intense emotional pressure I heaped upon my staff, I will never apologize for bringing loved ones back to their families, loved ones who, without these new technologies, would forever remain nameless.

My decisions to embrace universal mitochondrial typing and SNP testing were controversial. I've often asked myself: If I had it to do over again, given the same circumstances, would I make the same decisions? My honest response is yes. I might approach some problems differently, manage my resources better and more efficiently, be more staunch in my dealing with people, stay more on top of the many areas I neglected, but my basic decision to search for new technological approaches would not change.

I certainly did not do this alone. While many of my colleagues disagreed with my approach, they all, every one, backed me and helped pull me through the morass of technological data and issues that sprung up like weeds in a garden. Without the scientists on the Kinship and Data Analysis Panel, those in the private sector (the Bode Technology Group, Myriad Genetics, Celera Genomics, and Orchid Biosciences), governmental agencies (FBI, New York State Police, National Institute of Justice, National Institutes of Health, NIST, NCBI), and public forensic laboratories (the New York State Police and, of course, the OCME), I doubt we would have been as successful.

Still, the burden fell squarely on my shoulders. Mainly, help came from my most valuable resource—my staff. They pulled me through. I've mentioned their names, explained their roles, and illustrated how they went about their work for more than three years, even as outsiders forgot they were there. Truthfully, without them, many families would never have their loved ones. They are the true heroes of the identification work. Each of them worked tirelessly until I finally had to draw a line and force them to move on; to pause, as Chuck Hirsch likes to say.

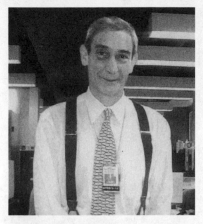

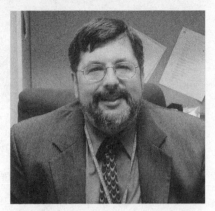

As chief medical examiner for the City of New York, Charles "Chuck" Hirsch had ultimate responsibility for identifying those who died at the World Trade Center and for returning their remains to the families. *(Photo by Carole Meyers)*

Howard Baum was my deputy director of the OCME DNA lab. *(Photo by Matt Benintendo)*

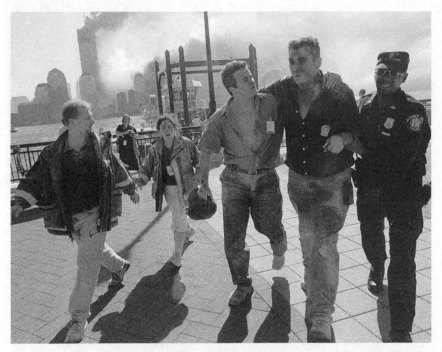

Ralph Ristenbatt, Amy Mundorff, Mark Desire, and Brian Gestring in Jersey City after they were nearly killed in the collapse of the first tower on September 11, 2001. *(Photo © 2001 Chip East/SIPA)*

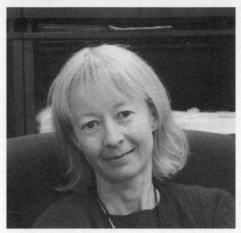

Mecki Prinz, assistant director in the OCME DNA laboratory. She was named director when I retired. (*Photo by Matt Benintendo*)

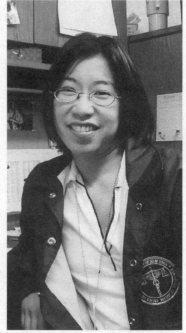

Elaine Mar, an OCME DNA laboratory criminalist, took over the second-floor DNA identification unit in December 2001. (*Photo by Carole Meyers*)

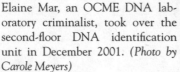

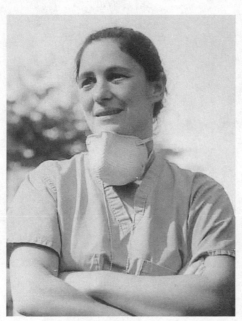

Amy Mundorff, the chief forensic anthropologist at the OCME, also supervised Memorial Park and was responsible for ensuring that the remains returned to the families were anthropologically correct. (*Photo © 2001, Richard Press*)

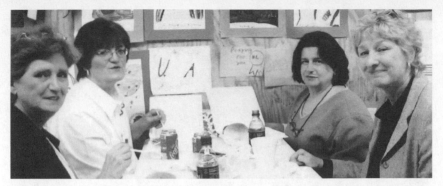

Grace Brugess, Joanne Valentine, Lorraine Kelly, and Ellen Borakove at Sal's Café. (*Photo by Carole Meyers*)

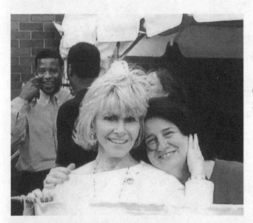

Carole Meyers and Lorraine Kelly at Sal's Café. (*Photo by Carole Meyers*)

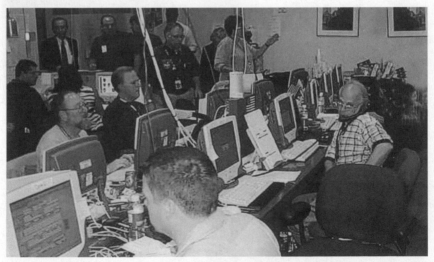

First-floor conference room at OCME connected into the WTC data center. (*Photo courtesy of Barbara Butcher*)

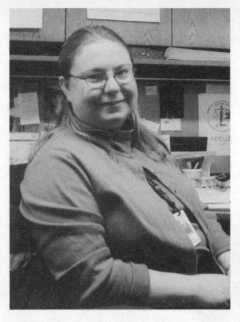

Noelle Umback, a criminalist in the OCME DNA lab. *(Photo by Carole Meyers)*

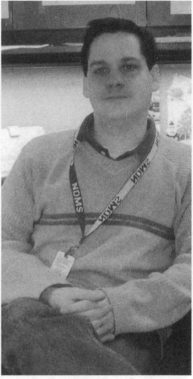

Mike Hennessey, a Gene Codes Forensics employee who worked under Elaine Mar in the second-floor DNA identification unit, devised the admin review process, and incorporated metadata into World Trade Center identifications. *(Photo by Carole Meyers)*

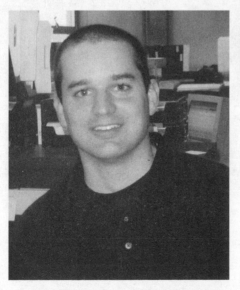

Erik Bieschke, a criminalist, was QA manager of the World Trade Center project. *(Photo by Matt Benintendo)*

Sheila Estacio Dennis, an OCME DNA laboratory criminalist, was a member of the World Trade Center special-projects team. *(Photo by Carole Meyers)*

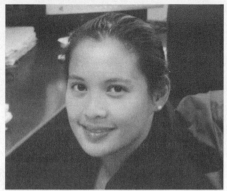

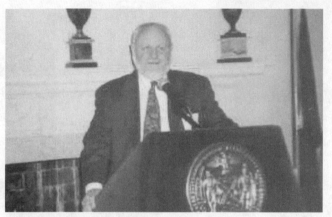

Dr. Robert Shaler at a breakfast at Gracie Mansion. *(Photo by Carole Meyers)*

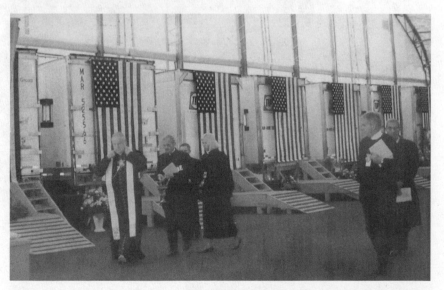

The refrigerated trailers at Memorial Park the day Cardinal Egan came to bless them. *(Photo by Carole Meyers)*

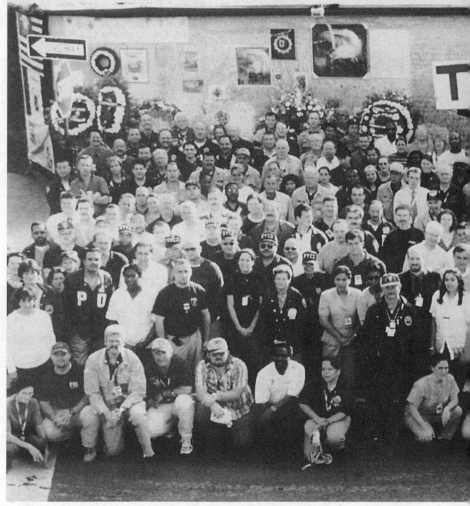

The staff of the New York City Office of Chief Medical Examiner along with members of federal, state, city, and volunteer organizations. (*Courtesy of Lorraine Kelly*)

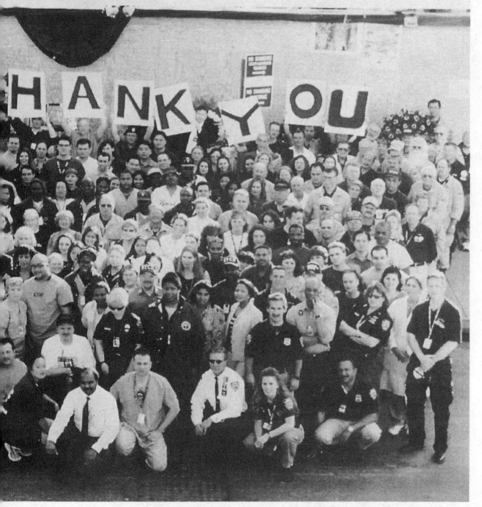

Medical Examiner
New York
eral, State, City,
Organizations

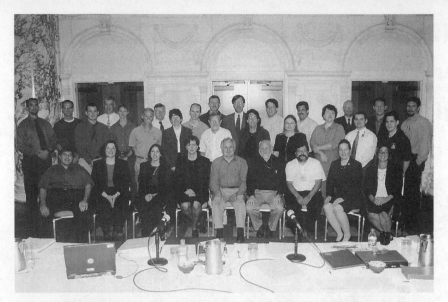

Attendees of the first KADAP meeting, New York, October 2001. (*Courtesy Amanda Sozer*)

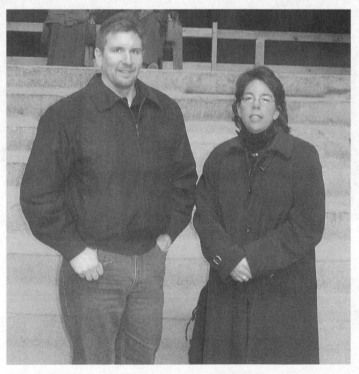

National Institute of Justice contractors and KADAP members Mandy Sozer and Steve Niezgoda. (*Courtesy Amanda Sozer*)

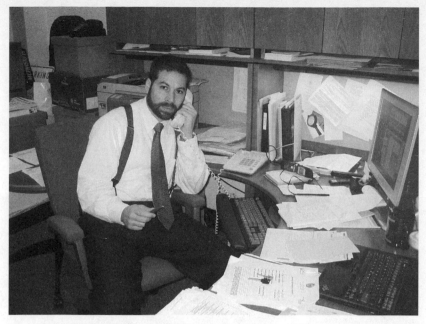

Shiya Ribowsky, Deputy Director Medicolegal Investigations. (*Courtesy Shiya Ribowsky*)

CAST OF CHARACTERS

Dwight Adams: director, FBI lab.

Mark Adams: professor, Case Western Reserve University; a Celera VP who replaced Rhonda Roby for the World Trade Center work.

Michael Baden: forensic pathologist, New York State Police and former chief medical examiner for the City of New York.

Jeanine Baiche: scientist, Orchid Biosciences, Dallas, Texas.

Howard Baum: deputy director, OCME DNA Lab.

Tracy Beeson: Gene Codes Forensics.

Erik Bieschke: criminalist, QA manager of the World Trade Center project; currently working in the molecular genetics division of the OCME DNA laboratory.

Todd Bille: assistant laboratory manager, special projects, Bode Technology Group.

David Boyd: Department of Homeland Security, previously of the National Institute of Justice.

Charles Brenner: OCME consultant, developed DNAView.

Tom Brondolo: OCME deputy commissioner, personnel, IT, procurement, for the World Trade Center work, responsible for IT operations and procurement.

Barry Brown: CODIS manager at the FBI during the World Trade Center work.

Zoran Budimlija: criminalist, OCME, and supervisor of special projects.

Bruce Budowle: research scientist, FBI and KADAP member.

Michele Buffolino: lost her mother, Rita Blau, during the World Trade Center attacks.

Pasquale "Pat" Buffolino: director, Nassau County Medical Examiner's Office DNA laboratory; was an assistant director in the OCME DNA laboratory during the early part of the World Trade Center work. He is not related to Michele.

Barbara Butcher: director, investigations; she replaced Dave Schomburg in 2004.

John Butler: a NIST scientist and KADAP member; he conceived the concept of miniplexes and developed the "Big Mini."

Bill Callahan: New York State Police.

Howard Cash: president, Gene Codes Forensics.

Judy Cash: Gene Codes employee during early part of the World Trade Center work and KADAP member.

Theresa Caragine: criminalist, OCME DNA laboratory; supervised the validation work for the Phase I extractions of tissues using the IQ system and in the research for Phase II extractions of tissues; currently supervisor, OCME DNA laboratory low-copy-number laboratory.

Cartier Family: the family that lost James, an apprentice electrician, during the World Trade Center attacks. Patrick is James's father. Patrick, John, and Michael are his brothers; Jennie, Michele, and Marie, his sisters.

James Marcel Cartier: an apprentice electrician, he died during the World Trade Center attacks.

Patrick Cartier: James Cartier's father.

Chris Cave: scientist, the Bode Technology Group.

Ranajit Chakraborty: professor, University of Cincinnati, who reviewed the SNP validation work.

Joselyn Cherwnjawski: criminalist, OCME DNA laboratory; responsible for purchasing laboratory supplies and equipment for the World Trade Center work.

Dianne Christie: medical legal investigator, OCME.

Mark Dale: inspector, NYS Forensic Investigation Center (Duceman's boss); currently at the University of Albany as the acting director of its NERFI program. After leaving the state police, he was the director of the New York City Police Department crime laboratory.

Ugo DeBlasi: Celera CFO.

Lydia DeCastro: criminalist, OCME DNA laboratory, and the sixth-floor disaster team rotation supervisor.

Frank DePaolo: medical legal investigator, the OCME mass-disaster coordinator.

Lisa Palumbo Desire: OCME DNA laboratory criminalist; she was the DNA laboratory STR rotation supervisor for the World Trade Center work.

Mark Desire: criminalist, OCME DNA laboratory; he supervised the processing of personal effects and buccal swabs for the American Airlines Flight 587 crash and for the OCME-based World Trade Center work.

Joe DiZinno: assistant director, FBI laboratory.

Karen Dooling: assistant director, OCME DNA laboratory until December 2001; currently a scientist at the Nassau County, New York, Medical Examiner's DNA laboratory.

Bill Doyle: lost his son during the World Trade Center attacks; a Staten Island family representative and member of the family group Give Your Voice.

Barry Duceman: director, New York State Police Biological Sciences Laboratory at the Forensic Investigation Center, Albany.

Sheila Estacio Dennis: criminalist, OCME DNA laboratory, member of the World Trade Center special projects team.

Jenny Farrell: James Cartier's sister.

David Feldt: Gene Codes. He was the first to explain the concept of metadata to me.

Joanne Feliciano: medicolegal investigator, OCME; worked with Shiya Ribowsky on both the American Airlines Flight 587 and World Trade Center work.

Paul Ferrara: director, Virginia Bureau of Forensic Science.

Stephanie Fiore: medical examiner, OCME. No longer with the OCME.

Mark Flomenbaum: deputy chief medical examiner; now the chief medical examiner for the state of Massachusetts.

Lisa Forman: director, Investigative and Forensic Science, National Institute of Justice.

Ron Forney: chief forensic scientist, Royal Canadian Mounted Police.

Brian Gestring: criminalist, professor of forensic science, Pace University.

Bob Giles: manager, Orchid Biosciences, Dallas, Texas.

Richard Gould: professor of archaeology, Brown University; suggested that remains had been spread beyond the original search area.

Elliot Gross: OCME chief after Michael Baden.

Kecia Harris: criminalist, OCME DNA laboratory; worked for Elaine Mar in the second-floor DNA ID unit.

Sarah Hart: chief administrator, National Institute of Justice; was David Boyd's and Lisa Forman's boss.

Mike Hennessey: Gene Codes Forensics employee; worked under Elaine in the second-floor DNA ID unit; devised the administrative review process and incorporated metadata into World Trade Center identifications.

Ashie Henry: head secretary, OCME DNA laboratory.

John Hicks: director, Forensic and Victims Services at NYS Division of Criminal Justice Services.

Charles "Chuck" Hirsch: chief medical examiner for the City of New York; he was ultimately responsible for identifying those who died at the World Trade Center and for returning their remains to the families.

Charity Holland: Bode Technology Group scientist; performed mtDNA typing on World Trade Center remains and personal effects.

Mitchell Holland: director, Bode forensic laboratory; responsible for STR and mtDNA typing of the bones recovered from the World Trade Center and Staten Island landfill sites. He is Charity's husband.

Ed Huffine: ICMP; during the World Trade Center work, directed the DNA identification of those who died in Bosnia. He came to New York to demonstrate the software that was being developed by the ICMP for that work. Currently at the Bode Technology Group.

Brett Hutchinson: criminalist, OCME; currently works for the New Jersey State Police DNA laboratory.

Chris Kamnik: criminalist, OCME DNA laboratory.

Lorraine Kelly: responsible for purchasing all the supplies needed by OCME scientists, medical examiners, medicolegal investigators, and administrators for the World Trade Center work.

Benoit Leclair: developer of MDKAP; scientist, Myriad Genetics.

Jack Lynch and his wife, Cathleen: lost their firefighter son Michael in the World Trade Center attacks.

Kevin MacElfresh: president and co-founder, Bode Technology Group.

Elaine Mar: DNA laboratory criminalist, OCME; she replaced Karen Dooling in December 2001 and supervised the second-floor DNA ID unit.

Michele Martinez: criminalist, OCME DNA laboratory; her first day at the OCME DNA laboratory was September 10, 2001. She was assigned to the sixth-floor disaster team, where she worked until she was reassigned to the second-floor DNA ID unit; now working in the fashion industry in midtown Manhattan.

Arne Masibay: Promega sales representative; he called on September 12, 2001, and is the reason the World Trade Center work began using robotics and the Promega IQ extraction system.

Jim McMahon: superintendent, New York State Police.

Carole Meyers: forensic DNA analyst, OCME; worked in the second-floor DNA ID unit.

Teri Michaud: New York City OMB staff.

Amy Mundorff: chief forensic anthropologist, OCME; also supervisor of Memorial Park and responsible for ensuring that the remains returned to the families were anthropologically correct.

Gene Myers: vice president, Celera Genomics.

Randy Nagy: vice president, marketing, Bode Technology Group.

Bianca Nazzaurolo: criminalist, OCME DNA laboratory; a member of the original sixth-floor disaster team and part of the special projects group; currently teaches high school biology in New York City.

Anca Nicholson: criminalist, OCME DNA laboratory, worked on the second-floor DNA ID unit; currently working criminal cases in the DNA laboratory.

Steve Niezgoda: NIJ contractor; he came to the OCME in December 2001. I asked him to be the World Trade Center daily project manager; also a KADAP member.

Judy Nolan: ex–Gene Codes Forensics scientist and original KADAP member.

Cathy Ordonez: president, Celera Genomics, after Craig Venter left the company.

Tom Parsons: research scientist, AFDIL; an internationally recognized expert in mtDNA and KADAP member.

Mark Perlin: founder, Cybergenetics Corp and author of True Allele, an artificial-intelligence software program designed to evaluate STR data.

Mecki Prinz: assistant director, OCME DNA laboratory, she played a major role in the World Trade Center Phase II STR typing and kinship analysis; she also reviewed STR data and performed kinship analysis for the American Airlines Flight 587 work.

Elizabeth Pugh: NIH Human Genome Project, Johns Hopkins University, and KADAP member.

Larry Quarino: forensic science professor, Cedar Crest College; he initiated the quality-assurance program for the World Trade Center work.

Shiya Ribowsky: deputy director, Medicolegal Investigations, and responsible for World Trade Center identifications; currently, assistant director for IT at the OCME and consultant, *Law & Order.*

Ralph Ristenbatt: criminalist, OCME; supervisor, Medical Examiner's Scientific Assessment and Training Team (MESATT; now Forensic Analysis and Reconstruction Unit).

Rhonda Roby: forensic scientist, Applied Biosystems; in charge of Soaring Eagles at Celera Genomics and supervised the mtDNA typing for the World Trade Center work.

Dr. Saha: former chairperson, New York City Department of Health Institutional Review Board.

Marie Samples: assistant director, OCME DNA laboratory; she kept the regular casework on track during the World Trade Center work and reviewed STR data for the American Airlines Flight 587 work.

Kristin Schelling: DNA scientist, Biosciences Unit, New York State Police, Albany; during the World Trade Center work, she worked with Peter Wistort.

Richie Scherer: Mayor Rudolph Giuliani's director, Office of Emergency Management.

Dave Schomburg: director, Medicolegal Investigations; currently lives in the Poconos.

Jim Schumm: research scientist, Bode Technology Group; designed the Bodeplex miniplexes based on John Butler's concept of the "Big Mini."

Sarah Scott: OCME general counsel to the chief medical examiner during the World Trade Center work; currently living in Texas.

Steve Sherry: scientist, National Center for Biological Informatics.

Jennifer Simon: criminalist, OCME DNA laboratory; currently in Seattle, Washington.

Jennifer Smith: supervisor, FBI DNA lab in Washington, DC; currently detailed to the CIA.

John Snyder: New York State Police contractor responsible for the BEAST installation; currently with Gene Codes Forensics.

Amanda "Mandy" Sozer: National Institute of Justice contractor and KADAP coordinator.

Dan Stevelman: director, facilities maintenance, OCME.

Tim Stockwell: vice president, Celera Genomics.

Mark Stolorow: executive director, Orchid Biosciences, Germantown, Maryland.

Katie Sullivan: liaison with the World Trade Center families; she worked for Shiya Ribowsky before taking over the World Trade Center investigations unit.

Noelle Umback: criminalist, OCME DNA lab.

Joanne Valentine: procurement, OCME.

Raju Venkataram: director, IT, OCME.

Craig Venter: founder, Celera Genomics.

Anne Walsh: New York State Department of Health.

Peter Wistort: CODIS manager, Bioscienses Unit, New York State Police, Albany.

GLOSSARY

accession: the process by which remains (actually, any evidence) are accepted into the OCME or the DNA laboratory. This is also known as the chain of custody, the legal documentation of everyone who handled evidence, when evidence was brought to the laboratory or OCME, where it was stored, and when it left.

administrative review, admin review: the process of checking and rechecking metadata (non-DNA data) to ensure accuracy in associating a missing person to a remain or DM.

allele: a genetic marker that occupies a specific location, or locus, on a chromosome. We inherit one allele from each parent.

allelic dropout: the loss of an allele. In practice, this happens in two ways—from either degraded or limiting amounts of DNA. Degraded or limiting amounts of DNA cause a weak signal that either isn't reported by instrumentation because of cutoffs established by the laboratory or because the allele is missing altogether.

amelogenin gene: the gene that determines the sex of an individual.

amplicon: the DNA amplification product of the polymerase chain reaction, or PCR. A fragment of DNA whose size depends on the parameters of the PCR reaction. For the World Trade Center Phase III work, amplicons ranged between 55 and 218 base pairs. The normal size of amplification products used in Phase I testing ranged between 100 and 400 base pairs.

antemortem DNA: DNA of the missing people obtained from their personal effects such as a toothbrush, hairbrush, razor, biopsy, et cetera. It also refers to buccal (mouth) swabs from the blood relatives of missing people.

BEAST (Bar Coded Evidence Analysis Statistics and Tracking): a laboratory information system used to accession remains and put them into a database so they can be tracked and searched.

"Big Mini": the miniplex developed by Dr. John Butler of NIST.

blind proficiency test: a laboratory test in which results are blind to the laboratory taking the test. The purpose is to test a laboratory's ability to obtain reliable results under specific conditions. For the World Trade Center work, this exercise focused on the ability of labs to handle compromised tissue.

BodePlex: miniplexes developed by Dr. Jim Schumm of the Bode Technology Group based on the concept developed by Dr. John Butler; there were two Bodeplexes, 1 and 2.

buccal swab: mouth swab taken from a blood relative for a DNA sample.

Cambridge Reference Sequence (CRS): a consensus mitochondrial sequence of the D-loop sequence. The differences between the consensus sequence and an unknown mitochondrial sequence are put into a tabular format called a mitotype, which should match the maternal lineage of the family.

capillary electrophoresis: a technique used to separate DNA fragments of different sizes.

centrifuge tube: a conical tube. The one used for transporting World Trade Center samples from the morgue to the DNA laboratory was 50 milliliters in size.

CODIS (Combined DNA Index System): a national database of DNA profiles maintained by the FBI.

commingling: the mixing together of human remains.

core number: a sequential number assigned to remains as they were received into the OCME morgue.

data dump: receipt of electronic DNA data by the OCME from the outside labs.

direct matching: the process of matching DNA profiles from a human remain with that of a personal effect containing DNA from the missing person.

D-loop: a small region of the mitochondrial genome scientists use for body identifications. The D-loop varies greatly among individuals.

DM (Disaster Manhattan): prefix to a number assigned to each World Trade Center remain brought to the morgue.

DMORT (Disaster Mortuary Organized Response Team): a group of professionals who respond to mass disasters at the request of the state government; a division of the Department of Homeland Security.

DNA extraction: in the World Trade Center context, this refers to removing DNA from human remains, personal effects, buccal swabs, or other biological material.

DNA profile: DNA typing at several loci. A complete STR profile for input to CODIS should have successful results at 13 loci. In a WTC context, a DNA profile can include STRs and/or SNPs.

DNAView: the DNA parentage software package authored by Dr. Charles Brenner; arguably the most sophisticated commercially available parentage-kinship analysis available.

DQ (Disaster Queens): number prefix assigned to remains from the American Airlines Flight 587 crash in Queens, New York, on November 12, 2001.

electropherogram: the graphical output of STRs at each locus from an instrument called a genetic analyzer; commonly called the raw STR data.

forensic bone analysis: the analysis of DNA in bones.

fragmentation: the product of DNA decay that results from degradation. This typically happens in decomposing tissue.

genomic DNA: DNA that is located in the nucleus of the cell and is composed of the 46 chromosomes we normally think of as our genetic inheritance. It is a large linear molecule structured much like a twisted ladder. The rungs of the ladder are called base pairs, of which there are approximately 3 billion in humans. They contain DNA's four-letter universal code—ACTG—the sequence of which is individually unique, except in pairs of identical twins.

isoenzyme genetic markers: inherited enzyme markers that differ among people.

kinship analysis: an indirect method of identifying missing people using the genetic structure of the family. The DNA profile of the human remains must fit into the family genetic structure before an identification can be made.

LIMS (Laboratory Information Management System): software systems designed to streamline laboratory processes by eliminating manual chores. They range from simple evidence data storage and tracking systems to extremely complex programs that can interface with instruments, schedule work, prepare reports, develop management statistics, and track samples using bar codes.

linkage disequilibrium: the concept that certain alleles might be associated in the population. This might occur in neighboring alleles that are co-inherited and are tightly linked.

LISA: software used to match DNA profiles of human remains to personal effects and kinship samples. AFDIL used LISA to identify the September 11 Pennsylvania and Pentagon victims.

locus: a specific region of DNA.

mass spectrometry: technique that fragments molecules into component parts based on their structure; commonly used to ascertain the molecular structure of unknown molecules.

MDKAP (Mass Disaster Kinship Analysis Program): an Excel spreadsheet program that matched STR DNA profiles. Its kinship routines used pairwise comparison of alleles to link families. The program has been commercialized under the trade name of Bloodhound.

Memorial Park: the location on 30th Street in Manhattan at the OCME where World Trade Center and American Airlines Flight 587 remains were stored.

MESATT (Medical Examiner's Scientific Assessment and Training Team): now referred to as FARU (Forensic Analysis and Reconstruction Unit).

metadata: for mass-fatality events, this is the non-DNA data from all sources.

MFISys (Mass Fatality Identification System): pronounced *emphasis*; a software program written for the OCME by Gene Codes Forensics.

microcentrifuge tube: a conical tube used in DNA laboratory procedures. It typically holds 1.5 milliliters.

microtiter plate: a plastic tray molded to form individual wells. These are used by automated liquid-handling systems in simple, repetitive laboratory chores such as transferring a sample from one tube or tray to another tube or tray. Although a microtiter plate can hold anywhere from 48 to 1,536 samples, the most popular configuration is an 8 x 12-inch format of 96 individual samples.

middleware: software programs used as a "bridge" between other software programs.

miniplexes: a concept developed by Dr. John Butler using STR amplicons specifically designed to work with degraded DNA. The first applied to the World Trade Center work was the "Big Mini." Two miniplexes designed by Dr. Jim Schumm of the Bode Technology Group for the World Trade Center work were called Bodeplex 1 and 2.

mitotype: tabular formatting of the differences between the D-loop sequence and the Cambridge Reference Sequence. The mitotype should match the maternal lineage of the family.

MOS (Members of Service): these included members of the FDNY, NYPD, EMS, and Port Authority Police.

mtDNA: mitochondrial DNA; it is circular and located inside the mitochondria of a cell. It is maternally inherited and, while useful to track maternal lineage, it is not necessarily unique. Different from nuclear DNA, which is typically employed in forensic testing, it has been used to aid in identifying human remains.

P number: family tracking number assigned by the New York City Police Department at Family Assistance Centers.

Phase I testing: the first round of STR testing of the remains and personal effects of the World Trade Center victims. It employed conventional STR testing as it is employed in United States crime laboratories using the 13 CODIS loci used in the FBI's national DNA database.

Phase II testing: the systematic reextraction and analysis of remains and personal effects that had not yielded STR test results during Phase I testing sufficient to make an identification.

Phase III testing: employment of alternate DNA technologies, such as miniplexes and SNPs, and mtDNA in the World Trade Center DNA work.

postmortem DNA: DNA taken from postmortem tissue.

proteolytic enzymes: enzymes that specifically chew up proteins.

RFU (relative fluorescence unit): a measure of the amount of DNA being analyzed. Small RFUs indicate small amounts of DNA. The instrument used to analyze STRs is normally set to "recognize" STRs at a minimum number of RFUs. If the DNA being analyzed has a small amount of DNA and the RFUs are below the instrument's cutoff, the instrument will not "call," or record, it. In these instances, the data, although not lost, will not be reported.

RM (reported missing): prefix to a unique number, one for each person missing in the World Trade Center disaster, based on a classification system developed by Shiya Ribowsky. By consolidating each missing person's complicated numerical history into a single number, we were able to simplify the identification process.

serology: the study of bodily fluids.

signal intensity: peak height on an electropherogram, which is measured by an arbitrary scale measured in RFUs.

SNP (single nucleotide polymorphism): a variation at a single, specific DNA base pair, the smallest level of variation on the DNA molecule.

SP (State Police): prefix to a unique number assigned to the DNA extract from a personal effect. It related to a WDI number, to which a family name was attached.

STR (short tandem repeat): biological markers inherited from our parents that vary widely among people. Testing for an STR at each of up to 16 different regions of the DNA results in a virtually unique DNA profile, referred to as an STR profile. The 13 loci form the basis of the FBI's national DNA database, CODIS. STRs in identical twins are the same. STR testing is the foundation of forensic testing worldwide.

TSNPs (threshold SNPs): SNPs characterized by their ability to resist allelic dropout when the amounts of DNA become limiting. When they fail, the entire SNP type disappears, not just one of the two alleles. We used them as first-stage markers to ascertain the reliability of SNP data when we were working with partial SNP profiles.

validation: scientific testing required to prove that a method is reliable for its intended purpose. Validation for the World Trade Center testing procedures showed that the methods we used gave reliable results with badly degrading DNA.

VIP (Victim Information Profile): a seven-page questionnaire designed by DMORT and completed by those reporting a missing person. For the World Trade Center work, it was filled out by hand at a Family Assistance Center (FAC) and then transcribed into a database. It contains information about the missing person (work history, jewelry, clothing, scars, tattoos, etc.), contact information for the family, and relationships of family members for antemortem DNA collection.

virtual DNA profile: a single STR profile constructed from two or more partial profiles after multiple testing of the same DM or personal effect. If the data is combined appropriately, it creates a DNA profile composite, a virtual profile.

WDI number (World Trade Center DNA identification number): a unique number assigned to each family by the New York State Police. Each family supposedly had a single one, but because families came to the Family Assistance Centers more than once, families often had multiple WDI numbers.

World Trade Center CODIS; WTC CODIS: a stand-alone CODIS network set up by the FBI at the Forensic Information Center in Albany specifically for the World Trade Center work. This network was not connected to the FBI's national DNA database, CODIS.

ACKNOWLEDGMENTS

There are innumerable people who share credit for this work. My wife, Fran Gdowski, not only stood by me throughout the WTC work and encouraged me to write this book but also worked in the morgue on weekends. To this day, she is still devastated by the events of September 11. My children, Christie and TJ, cared for and encouraged and stood by me. Dr. Charles Hirsch, the chief medical examiner, set our ethical standards and had faith in me. The OCME staff, especially the forensic scientists in the Department of Forensic Biology, dedicated their lives to the families and made our successes possible. The forensic scientists at the New York State Police, Myriad Genetics, Celera Genomics, Orchid Biosciences, and the Bode Technology Group ensured our success. Shiya Ribowsky became a friend and confidant and worked with me throughout. He and Katie Sullivan and the medicolegal investigators worked tirelessly with my staff to return missing loved ones to their families. Amy Mundorff managed Memorial Park and became a close friend and confidante. Also, many unselfishly volunteered their time. For this, I thank the scientists at the New Jersey State Police and the medical students at Columbia and New York universities. Thanks to the program engineers at Gene Codes Forensics, who wrote MFISys; Benoit Leclair for MDKAP; and Charles Brenner for DNAView. Thanks to Lisa Forman for the Kinship and Data Analysis Panel, the KADAP, for their expertise and guidance. My friends and colleagues—you know who you are—supported me during those chaotic times and then encouraged me to write this book. Liz Stein, my editor, conceived the idea of a book and then guided me through the process, giving me the opportunity to publicly thank my colleagues. Finally, there are the families who empathized with us and encouraged us throughout.

INDEX

Page numbers in *italics* refer to figures, tables, and photographs

ABOUT THE AUTHOR

Robert C. Shaler was the director of the Forensic Biology Department of the Office of the Chief Medical Examiner of New York City from 1990 until his retirement in 2005. He is currently professor of biochemistry and molecular biology and director of the Forensic Science Program at Pennsylvania State University. He divides his time between State College, Pennsylvania, and Flemington, New Jersey.